Nursing Leadership and Management

HOW TO ORDER THIS BOOK

BY PHONE: 877-500-4337 or 717-290-1660, 9AM–5PM Eastern Time

BY FAX: 717-509-6100

BY MAIL: Order Department
DEStech Publications, Inc.
439 North Duke Street
Lancaster, PA 17602, U.S.A.

BY CREDIT CARD: American Express, VISA, MasterCard, Discover

BY WWW SITE: http://www.destechpub.com

Nursing Leadership and Management
The Advanced Practice Role

Edited by

Denise M. Korniewicz, Ph.D., RN, FAAN

Assessment Technologies Institute Nursing Education
Ascend Learning

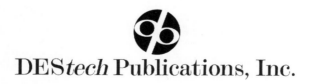

DES*tech* Publications, Inc.

Nursing Leadership and Management

DEStech Publications, Inc.
439 North Duke Street
Lancaster, Pennsylvania 17602 U.S.A.

Printed in the United States of America
10   9   8   7   6   5   4   3   2   1

Main entry under title:
    Nursing Leadership and Management: The Advanced Practice Role

A DEStech Publications book
Bibliography: p.
Includes index p. 193

Library of Congress Catalog Card No. 2015904000
ISBN No. 978-1-60595-158-4

Table of Contents

Preface

Nursing Leadership and Management: The Advanced Practice Role is the result of working with superb advanced practice professionals in clinical practice settings. Often, these excellent clinicians need additional leadership skills that can assist them in the everyday management and leadership positions that are continuously developing in our changing healthcare system. Advanced practice professional roles include nurses, physical therapists, pharmacists and other health professionals who are obtaining their terminal professional degrees such as the doctorate in nursing practice (DNP), doctorate of physical therapy (DPT), the doctorate in occupational therapy (DOT) or the doctorate of pharmacology (PharmD.). As a result, most educational programs integrate this content but do not provide specific examples or discuss the types of leadership issues that these professionals may encounter. The content of this book attempts to provide advanced practice professionals with the practical approaches needed to be an effective leader in clinical settings. Thus, the purpose of this book is to provide the scientific underpinnings for effective leadership in clinical practice settings and to assist interdisciplinary health professionals with the skills necessary to transform our healthcare organizations.

There are many leadership books available for healthcare professionals, however, most review the basic concepts of leadership such as those associated with the views of business or management. However, the approach offered in this book reflects case studies and references associated with interdisciplinary and inter-professional leadership encounters that are realistic cases that occur in clinical practice settings. Each chapter will present a case study depicting the concepts reflective of a clinical issue that involves the application of leadership principles that are necessary to solve the problem.

The book has been divided in six major themes: (1) scientific principles of leadership; (2) understanding leadership in traditional & non-traditional healthcare settings; (3) promoting leadership for quality patient care; (4) developing clinical scholarship; (5) transforming healthcare and (6) inter-professional models of healthcare. Within each chapter, a case study is presented to assist the reader with critical decision making skills needed for effective and safe clinical practice. The ability for the advanced practice professional to acquire increased leadership skills within the clinical practice setting provides a solid foundation for improving patient care. This book provides a practical approach to the application of leadership principles while systematically presenting the content needed for skilled leadership in the clinical setting.

The author's deep gratitude is expressed to all the chapter authors who provided creative case studies and important content for this book. A thanks goes to numerous friends and colleagues who facilitated this effort and provided critique of the content. A special thanks goes to my colleagues Chris Harsell, Jackie Roberts, and Maridee Shogren who were wonderful at assisting with the initial content to understand what newly prepared DNP nurse practitioners needed to be successful clinical leaders. Finally, the constant encouragement of my sister Sandy Korniewicz who always provides indirect encouragement to complete the project and my adopted sister, Margaret Brack, whose positive support helped me to complete this endeavor.

DENISE KORNIEWICZ

List of Contributors

Mary E. Asher DNP, RN, CNS, CPAN
School of Nursing and Health Sciences
University of Miami
Coral Gables, FL

Christianne Fowler DNP, GNP-BC
School of Nursing
Old Dominion University
Norfolk, VA

Tina Haney DNP, CNS
School of Nursing
Old Dominion University
Norfolk, VA

Christine C. Harsell DNP, ANP-BC
College of Nursing & Professional Disciplines
University of North Dakota
Grand Forks, ND

Jacqueline Roberts DNP, FNP-BC, AOCNP
College of Nursing & Professional Disciplines
University of North Dakota
Grand Forks, ND

Carolyn M. Rutledge PHD., FNP-BC
Director, Doctor of Nursing Practice Program
School of Nursing
Old Dominion University
Norfolk, VA

Judy Seltzer MS, BSN, BN, CNOR
Surgical Clinical Director, Corporate Accounts
Molnlycke Health Care
Norcross, GA

Laurel S. Shepherd PHD., RN
Educational & Accreditation Consultant
Norfolk, VA

Maridee Shogren DNP, CNM
College of Nursing & Professional Disciplines
University of North Dakota
Grand Forks, ND

Jeanne H. Siegel PHD., ARNP
Educational Consultant
Miami, FL

Joanna Sikkema DNP, ANP-BC, FAHA, FPCNA
College of Nursing & Professional Disciplines
University of North Dakota
Grand Forks, ND

Mary M. Wyckoff PHD., NNP-BC, ACNP, BC, FNP-BC, CCNS, CCRN, FAANP
Neonatal Intensive Care
University of California, Davis
Clitical Care Clinical Consultant
Sacramento, California

Exploring Leadership Theories for Advanced Practice Nurses

JEANNE H. SIEGEL PHD., ARNP
DENISE M. KORNIEWICZ PHD., RN, FAAN

The Chapter 1 case study demonstrates current perspectives about leadership theory and focuses on the integration of general leadership principles with the applied clinical sciences, emphasizing the advanced practice healthcare professional.

Case Presentation

Caroline Smart DNP, CNS, RN was a hospital nursing educator until her recent graduation from a Doctor of Nursing Practice Program. Upon graduation, the vice president promoted her to the position of Director of Medical Surgical Nursing Division. This division included a 45-bed medical telemetry floor, a 60-bed telemetry surgical floor, and a 32-bed step down Medical/Surgical ICU. Caroline was excited about the promotion but knew she would have a steep learning curve. She was delighted to discover that each of these units had an assistant director who was responsible for the staffing and day-to-day operations. Caroline would be responsible for budgets, hiring and firing decisions, quality assurance, purchasing, and employee evaluations.

The vice president did have one immediate concern: there had been numerous complaints about quality of patient care (patient complaints), low staff morale, high call out rates, and difficulty recruiting new staff. The hospital had to bring on a small number of agency nurses to meet the demands of these units. This agency was a tremendous financial drain on the hospital and it could not continue. Carolyn was given 6 months to evaluate the units to determine the root cause of the problem and take corrective action.

1

Caroline's leadership experience so far had been centered on a much smaller scale as a charge nurse and directing educational endeavors.

Caroline recalled how all of her nursing instructors emphasized the need to perform a complete assessment of a situation before determining the cause of the problem or taking any action. She concluded that this advice would also work in the management field. Her plan consisted of observation of the day-to-day operations of each of her units prior to sharing her concerns with her staff. She made herself visible on each shift, participated in patient care, assisted in decision-making, and got to know the staff of each unit. Caroline also had the opportunity to get informal feedback from many of her staff. She discovered that several other key nursing personnel were considering leaving, characterizing the units as "dysfunctional and under staffed" and without leadership to intervene on their behalf. Caroline had never asked what caused the prior director to leave, but she was certainly starting to get the picture.

After 3 weeks of collecting evidence of the issues that existed on each of her units, Caroline found the following:

1. 45-bed medical telemetry floor—Despite having designated day and night assistant directors and charge nurses that had been with the organization for many years, no one was really in charge. The assistant director/charge nurse could be found at the main desk or in the employees lounge on the phone. They made shift and new admission assignments, rarely taking patients of their own. They did not make rounds to evaluate patients' progress. Occasionally, they were asked to see a patient related to a complaint, but there was never evidence of a resolution. The hospital had a policy and documentation system for administrative unit rounds on each patient and each unit for every shift. No documentation could be found that this was being completed. New registered nurse staff (new graduates and new hires) did not appear to use the designated nurse leaders as resources. This explained some physician complaints about "a bunch of novice nurses running the show." Additionally, the nursing administration had received multiple family complaints about the lack of response to call lights, pain medicine requests, and unanswered calls at the nursing station.

2. 60-bed telemetry surgical floor—Caroline spent a lot of her time on this floor, making rounds and working beside the nursing staff. The day and night assistant directors, though only 3 years out from

graduation, appeared to be committed to the unit and to be delivering good patient care. The staff recently began a pilot to do self-scheduling and was trying to develop a modified self-governance model. Unfortunately, there was a serious divide between the registered nurses (RNs) and the nursing assistants (NAs) leading to poor delivery of care. Complaints of delayed call light responses and increased falls was a major concern. Both the RNs and NAs blamed the other group to be at fault for the increase in patient falls. Staff turnover was high, with most new hires leaving before their first year anniversary. There was an obvious need for team building on this unit.

3. 32-bed step down Medical/Surgical ICU—This unit had the strongest mix of nurses. Almost all the nurses had Baccalaureate or Masters Degrees in Nursing or other fields. The nurses had a minimum of 5 years of experience. The staffing ratio was 4:1, with nursing assistants available for the more difficult physical care of patients. It did not take long for Caroline to realize that there was no teamwork or cohesion on this unit. The designated charge nurses had given up trying to lead or develop the staff. Every nurse that worked on the unit believed that their view was the correct one. They continued to practice nursing the way they learned it. Discussions of policy, procedure, evidenced-based practice, and team consensus did not exist.

Caroline had to develop a plan, but needed to prioritize the issues. Even though each of the units had problems, there were common themes across all three. First, there was inconsistent or no strong leadership on each of the units. She had nurses in leadership positions that were not well versed in leadership skills or competencies. With the permission of the VP of nursing, she choose to educate and develop their skills, and then if necessary, replace the leaders who were unwilling or unable to learn and change. To begin the transformation, Caroline developed educational meetings to educate all staff about the definition of leadership, theories of leadership, and how leadership affects healthcare outcomes (based on evidence). In addition, she held focus groups with staff to obtain input about how to resolve the individual unit issues and monitor the progress from within. She began team-building strategies by using the "Core Competencies for Interprofessional Collaborative Practice" (AACN, AACOM, AACP, ADE, and AMC 2011). The VP supported the idea and was interested in using the program system-wide, if the results were positive.

ESSENTIAL PRINCIPLES OF LEADERSHIP

There are several concepts that need to be explored to develop advance practice nurse (APN) leaders. These principles include an understanding of the definitions of leadership, characteristics of effective leaders and the scientific theories that undergird the principles of leadership. Because the healthcare environment is undergoing massive change, APNs will need to develop additional leadership skills that encompass changes in the clinical environment and will need to provide accountability for quality patient care. Often, APNs are clinical experts but lack proficiency at managing clinical staff. Perhaps one way to further develop the skills necessary for APNs to become the future leaders of population-based clinical care is to provide a leadership framework that balances the theory and application of leadership principles.

Caroline recalled how all of her nursing instructors emphasized the need to perform a complete assessment of a situation before determining the cause of the problem or taking any action. She concluded that this advice would also work in the management field.

Defining Leadership

The literature has a cadre of definitions that have been used to define leadership. Daft (2008) has defined leadership as consisting of six essential elements: influence, intention, personal responsibility, change, shared purpose, and followers. Others have defined leadership as the art or process of influencing people using interpersonal skills that help others achieve their highest potential (Weihrich and Koontz 2005; Sullivan and Garland 2010; ANA 2014) (Table 1.1). Further, the ability to be an effective leader within an organization requires skills associated with collaboration, diversity, empowerment and ethical purpose.

Leaders are often described as powerful, influential, charismatic, dynamic, innovative, clever, autocratic, innovative, and intelligent (Curtis *et al.* 2011). In a recent study (Winston and Patterson 2006), a review of the leadership literature showed that leadership definitions consisted of over 90 variables and focused only on isolated descriptors such as process or behaviors versus encompassing attributes that define the whole of leadership. Reed and Winston (2005) further define leadership as an integrative approach that focuses on the use of critical thinking skills, interpersonal communication, and the ability to be an active listener who can assist others in positive change within an organization.

TABLE 1.1. *Definitions of Leadership.*

Leadership Reference	Definition
Weihrich, H. and H. Koontz. 2005. *Management a Global Perspective,* 11th ed., McGraw Hill, Singapore.	"Leadership is defined as influence, that is, the art or process of influencing people so that they will strive willingly and enthusiastically toward the achievement of group goals."
Winston, B.E. and K. Patterson. 2006. An Integrative Definition of Leadership. *International Journal of Leadership Studies 1,* 2, pp. 6–66.	"A leader is one or more people who selects, equips, trains, and influences one or more follower(s) who have diverse gifts, abilities, and skills and focuses the follower(s) to the organization's mission and objectives causing the follower(s) to willingly and enthusiastically expend spiritual, emotional, and physical energy in a concerted coordinated effort to achieve the organizational mission and objectives."
Sullivan, E.J. and G. Garland. 2010. *Practical Leadership and Management in Nursing.* Pearson Education Limited; Harlow.	"Leadership involves the use of interpersonal skills to influence others to accomplish a specific goal."
American Nurse Association (ANA). 2014. *Leadership Definition.* Retrieved May 19, 2014. http://www.nursingworld.org/Main-MenuCategories/ThePracticeofProfessionalNursing/Leadership	"Leaders do more than delegate, dictate, and direct. Leaders help others achieve their highest potential. At ANA, we empower nurses to be professional, competent leaders in healthcare. Through a variety of educational and advocacy activities, our work increases the leadership capacity of nurses to advance health and lead change."

Her plan consisted of observation of the day-to-day operations of each of her units prior to sharing her concerns with her staff. She made herself visible on each shift, participated in patient care, assisted in decision-making, and got to know the staff of each unit. Caroline also had the opportunity to get informal feedback from many of her staff. She discovered that several other key nursing personnel were considering leaving, characterizing the units as "dysfunctional and under staffed" and without leadership to intervene on their behalf. Caroline had never asked what caused the prior director to leave, but she was certainly starting to get the picture.

Leaders have a broad range of expectations and roles. Often the roles of a leader have been described as a change agent, problem solver, influencer, advocate, teacher, forecaster (long term view), facilitator, risk taker, idea originator, challenger, and communicator (Curtis *et al.* 2011; Marquis and Huston 2009). Other characteristics of leaders include intelligence, knowledge, judgment, independence, personable, adaptable, creative, and innovative. However, the leader within the organization may or may not be part of the formal organizational structure, rather, they may use their influence to obtain power and authority to influence others within the organization. What is important about the role of the leader is how their role is perceived within in the organization and what impact they may have on the overall operations within the system. APNs need to be cognizant of their role within a healthcare organization in order to be an effective leader.

Effective Leadership

Research has shown that effective leaders achieve results by influencing, motivating, and inspiring employees over whom they may or may not have direct supervision (Cummings 2008). In fact, leaders that focused on relationships (transformational, supportive, considerate) were associated with higher nurse job satisfaction and increased retention. Noneffective leaders were more inclined to focus on tasks versus the individual employee that resulted in low morale, decreased job satisfaction, and increased staff turnover.

> Caroline spent a lot of her time on this floor, making rounds and working beside the nursing staff. The day and night assistant directors, though only 3 years out from graduation, appeared to be committed to the unit and to be delivering good patient care. The staff recently began a pilot to do self-scheduling and was trying to develop a modified self-governance model. Unfortunately, there was a serious divide between the RNs and the NAs leading to poor delivery of care.

Guyton (2012) proposed nine principles that contributed to effective leadership. These principles were proposed to guide clinical nurse leaders and were targeted at leading clinical staff (Table 1.2). APNs could readily adapt these leadership principles when developing an action plan to improve patient care outcomes. For example, by adapting a culture of accountability for patient care and providing evidence-based guidelines, APNs can provide the framework for safe clinical care while increasing both patient and clinical staff satisfaction.

Leadership Versus Management

Marquis and Huston (2009) have observed that there remains some confusion about the relationship between leadership and management. This relationship continues to prompt debate with some viewing leader-

TABLE 1.2. *Principles of Successful Nursing Leadership (Guyton 2012).*

Principle of Leadership	Action or Outcome
Commitment to excellence	Commitment to excellence begins with the leader.
Measure the important things	Identifies the need to measure patient and employees' satisfaction; quality of care; your employee's progress, unit growth, and development; and the unit's financial well being.
Build a culture around service	Reinforce the need for your staff to appreciate patients and families as customers.
Create and develop leaders	Leaders have a professional obligation to develop future leaders from within their ranks. The benefit to developing clinical nurse leadership is the ability for the unit to run when the senior leader is not present.
Focus on employee satisfaction	Employee satisfaction leads to employee retention. Focus on establishing an ongoing relationship with your employees.
Build individual accountability	Hold all employees responsible for their role/responsibilities within an organization.
Align behaviors with goals and values	Consistent behavioral standards that align with the organizational values, mission, and standards should be enforced.
Communicate on all levels	Communication should be based on an interdisciplinary framework.
Recognize and reward success	A system/program of ongoing recognition and rewards will reinforce the employees' excellence.

ship as one of many skills a manager should possess. Opposing scholars maintain that leadership requires more skills than management. Others argue that management's purpose is one of control and maintaining the status quo, whereas the leader empowers others, inspires innovation, and challenges traditional practice while motivating followers to a common goal (Curtis *et al.* 2011). The two roles are not necessarily exclusive. If a manager can guide, direct, inspire, and motivate they can also lead (Marquis and Huston 2009). Alternatively, leadership without the ability to manage, if in a management role, can also lead to a disaster.

Caroline Smart DNP, CNS, RN was a hospital nursing educator until her recent graduation from a Doctor of Nursing Practice Program. Upon graduation, the vice president promoted her to the position of Director of Medical Surgical Nursing Division. This division included a 45-bed medical telemetry floor, a 60-bed telemetry surgical floor, and a 32-bed step down Medical/Surgical ICU.

APNs are asked to take on added responsibilities within a health-care organization once they obtain their terminal degree (DNP). Often they are assigned to a position and title within the organization (Marquis and Huston 2009) and are asked to manage one or more units. They usually have delegating authority over both willing and unwilling subordinates (Curtis *et al.* 2011; Marquis and Huston 2009). By definition, a nursing leader innovates, inspires, guides, and challenges. Often, APNs are new to a management position and must rely on their clinical experience to develop the skills necessary to manage clinical staff members. Blending the characteristics of a good leader and the attributes of a skilled manager can challenge APNs as they make the transition from providing individual primary care service to providing leadership associated with the overall improvement of patient outcomes within a healthcare organization. Thus, the role of the APN is expanded to beyond that of a direct patient care provider to a supervisor of population-based healthcare by monitoring the work of other clinical staff members.

GENERAL THEORIES OF LEADERSHIP

The desire to develop a theory of leadership that simplifies the conditions that result in exceptional leaders has led to the development of a large number of theories across multiple disciplines. In nursing, APNs are expected to expand their roles as leaders in administration, education, and clinical practice. Today, APNs are challenged to incorporate leadership theories across clinical agencies in order to meet the future needs of healthcare providers and patients. However, the theory and practice of leadership has been developed from other disciplines and applied to the discipline of nursing.

What makes a great leader? Are leaders born with the traits necessary to lead under a variety of circumstances? Can leadership be taught? Are leadership qualities something you are born with? Does it help to read a plethora of books to develop leadership qualities? These questions have generated several theories associated with leadership and have been classified into categories ranging from the historical great man theories to the more contemporary leadership theories of the twenty-first century. The adaptation and use of a leadership theory by APNs as clinical experts depends on the type of position held within the organization as well as the philosophy and mission of the healthcare system.

Spector (2006a) categorized leadership theories in terms of approaches such as trait, behavioral, contingency/situational, and leader/member (Table 1.3). In general, most leadership theories can be categorized as one of these leadership styles. Depending on the definitions of each of these approaches and the expected outcomes associated with the leadership style, the theoretical underpinnings of each have historically developed as organizations have matured and changed within society.

The *trait approach* is concerned with personal traits that contribute to effective leadership. These include the Great Man Theory and Trait

TABLE 1.3. Types of Leadership Theories.

Leadership Theory	Era	Definition
Great Man (Boden 1994)	1930–1940	Proposes that great men are born, not made, leading to the belief that great leaders will arise when there is a great need (Bolden *et al.*, 2003). This theory has since fallen out of favor. Scholars attempted to identify characteristics of great leaders that were based on the prevailing leaders of the day who were usually male and from the upper classes.
Trait/Behavioral (Taylor 2009)	1940–1980	A softer version of the Great Man Theory, it assumes that certain inherent traits and qualities make an individual better suited to a leadership role. These traits are generally described as personality or behavior characteristics that are shared by current or previous leaders.
Contingency/Situational (Taylor 2009)	1950–1980	Contingency theories are situational by their very nature. There is no one leadership style, quality, or trait that is best for all situations. The emphasis is on the factors that affect a particular situation. This theory chooses to focus on the environment that may influence the situation and that the ability to lead is contingent on the situation, the leader, and the follower. Situational-contingency theories do not recognize any one leadership approach. Fundamental to the theory is that different circumstances will require different types of leadership. Therefore, leaders may be effective in one situation and unable to lead in another.
Leader/Member exchange/ Transformational (Cherry 2014)	1970–today	The focus is on the relationships formed between the leader and their followers as being of critical importance (Boden *et al.* 2003). A transformational leader will motivate and inspire individuals by facilitating group members to see the importance of the goal at hand. Transformational leaders concentrate on the performance of group members, encouraging each member to fulfill his potential.

Theories that were popular until the mid-1940s. The *behavioral approach*, popular from 1940 to 1980, explores leadership from the perspective of the leader by examining the leader behaviors. Examples of the behavioral approach of leadership include those identified by Lewin (1951) and White (1960). The *contingency approach*, prevalent from 1950 to 1980, is based on Fielder's contingency theory and path-goal theory. This theory suggests that leadership is about the interaction between the leader, his behavior, and the situation. The *Leader-Member Exchange Approach* emerged in the 1970s and is referred to as charismatic or transformational leadership (Table 1.3). In fact, the term transformational leadership is still in use today and is focused on the relationship between the leader and the followers.

Other general theories of leadership include *participative* and *transactional*. Participative theory suggests that the ideal leadership style is to take into account the input of other stakeholders. The leader encourages participation and input from the group and its members feel important, and therefore committed to the process (Taylor 2009). *Transactional* theories are management styles of the role of supervisors in an organization and group performance (Cherry 2014). The theoretical foundation is based on rewards and punishment (Bolden *et al.* 2003). For example, businesses frequently use managerial theory by rewarding employees (money or rewards) who are successful, and conversely, reprimanding (punishing) employees that fail.

Most recently, *transformational leadership* has become widely accepted within organizations since the leader subscribes to high ethical and moral standards (Cherry 2014; Taylor 2009). There is an emphasis on the empowerment of followers, building a shared vision, and encouraging participation and motivation. Transformational theoretical models assert that individual members will follow leaders who inspire them. Transformational leadership qualities include vision, ability to inspire, trust, sharing a bond, and empowering others (Curtis *et al.* 2011). Studies based on the use of transformational leadership theory have demonstrated positive outcomes when compared to transactional leadership styles. In one study, there was a strong positive correlation to leaders' extra effort, leadership satisfaction, and effectiveness in the leaders demonstrating transformational leadership characteristics and that it was a predictor of leadership outcomes (Casida and Parker 2001).

CONTEMPORARY NURSING LEADERSHIP THEORIES

In the current healthcare environment, nursing leaders need to be prepared to respond to the ever changing needs and demands for quality nursing care. Nurse leaders of the twenty-first century may require more integrated models of leadership theory. Recent research by Stanley (2006b) has demonstrated that the use of transformational theory may be appropriate for administrative nurse leaders, but a different theoretical model may be needed for clinical leaders. Perhaps a combination of concepts from a variety of nursing leadership theories may be used to provide a framework for future APN leaders. These clinical nursing leadership theories have been identified as congruent/authentic, servant, principal agent, human/social capital, and emotional intelligence.

Congruent/authentic leadership theory suggests that leaders must be true to themselves, know their values, and act accordingly (Marquis and Huston 2009). According to Stanley (2006a), "Congruent leaders (clinical nurse leaders) are followed because there is a match between the leader's value and beliefs and their actions." The rapidly changing healthcare environment will require clinical leaders to learn new roles and develop new skills at an accelerated pace (Marquis and Huston 2009). Stanley (2006b) has suggested that the future of nursing leadership theory is beyond transformational leadership models because the clinical environment will be even more complicated than today's. Stanley (2006b) also suggests that the clinical environment of the future is unlike the other business environments, requiring a unique theory to guide its development. Congruent or authentic leadership requires leaders "to be matched (congruence) between the activities, actions, and deeds of the leader and the leader's values." APNs will be evaluated for their leadership skills within their work environment. For example, the application of this model will require the APN to integrate everyday clinical occurrence, staff knowledge and skills, and interdisciplinary team outcomes, and to apply their own beliefs in the clinical situation. The congruent/authentic leadership model provides a framework for APNs to adapt and to measure the overall quality of patient care based on their leadership style.

Servant leadership theory argues that in order to be a great leader, one needs to be a servant first (Greenleaf 1977). Although the premise of servant leadership theory was developed over 30 years ago, the theory continues to influence today's leaders. Greenleaf based his model on his observation that successful leaders lead in a different manner than traditional leaders. Recent work by Marquis and Huston (2009) suggested that servant leaders have 10 qualities that define their success. These attributes include listening on a deep level, truly understanding, being open minded, being comfortable dealing with complex issues, ambiguity, and paradoxes, the ability to involve all parties in challenging situations and requesting their input, being goal directed, demonstrating the ability to be servant, helper, and teacher first, then leader, thinking before acting, carefully choosing words, possessing foresight and intuition, and looking at the big picture, sensing relationships, and connections. The ability of the APN to incorporate some of the servant theory attributes into their leadership style will enhance their clinical management skills.

The *principal agent* leadership theory was derived from an economics model in the 1960s and was categorized as another interactive theory. The hallmark of this model is the belief that not all followers (called agents) are naturally motivated to support the best interest of the leader or employer (principal). This assumes that in order for the followers to perform, adequate incentives must be provided. Unfortunately, in most healthcare models there are little incentives provided for followers, thus the relationship between the principal (APN) and the agent (healthcare personnel) must be one that fosters compliance with the vision, mission, or goals of the principal. APNs who use this leadership theory may have to develop incentives for healthcare staff such as monetary rewards, promotion, employee recognition awards, or recognition by their peers. Additionally, APNs may influence management changes by adapting new ways to reward patient followers who adapt health compliance or incentives.

The *human capital* theory of leadership recognizes the need for individuals and organizations to invest in employees with the anticipation of future gains. Human capital is usually viewed as the collective education, knowledge, skills, and abilities of an entire group. Human capital theory assumes that these gains can be increased or improve productivity. Thus, longevity in the work place becomes a desirable outcome for valued employees. APNs who invest in employees who foster excellence in the healthcare environment understand that in the long term their initial investment of time, energy, or effort substantially pays off. For example, the motivational basis for providing tuition reimbursement to employees is for their advancement to benefit the organization at a later point in time. A second example in which APNs may influence patients is to invest in educating a diabetic patient about diet and exercise so that over time there is less cost in care because the patient may prevent further health deterioration. APNs familiar with the use of human capital leadership theory can apply these concepts within the clinical environment.

The *emotional intelligence* theory is defined as the ability to perceive emotions, facilitate thinking, and to analyze or understand the relationships of others to one's own emotions (Mayer *et al.* 2000). Studies have demonstrated that an emotionally intelligent nurse leader is an individual who can work in harmony with his/her thoughts and feelings and are able to better manage stress in the clinical environment (Freshwater and Stickley 2004). Furthermore, nurse leaders who have been high performers have had high emotional inteligence scores. Emotional intelligence has been correlated with improved retention, less burnout, and healthy workplace environments. Nurse managers who understand the concepts associated with emotional intelligence are proactive and problem-focused, thus their ability to facilitate less-stressful clinical environments promotes safer and better patient care.

APNs will experience a variety of leadership roles within the clinical area. Since the role of the APN is continuously changing, it is important for the clinical leader to be knowledgeable about the different leadership theories and their application to clinical practice. Despite the vast array of clinical practice settings and the divergent roles of the APN, the ultimate aim of leadership is to improve patient care outcomes. As APNs engage in a variety of leadership activities, their responsibilities and level of leadership abilities will increase. Therefore, it is important that the APNs are aware of their own limitations and continue to be willing to be effective patient care advocates.

SUMMARY POINTS

- APNs are effective leaders within the clinical environment.
- The application and understanding of leadership theories provide a conceptual framework for APNs who manage patient care.
- APNs must have an understanding of the difference between leadership and management.
- Some of the current leadership theories can be applied to the clinical area.

REFERENCES

American Nurse Association (ANA). 2014. *Leadership Definition.* Retrieved June 6, 2014. http://www.nursingworld.org/MainMenuCategories/ThePracticeofProfessionalNursing/Leadership

American Nurses Credentialing Center (ANCC), 2014. *Magnet Recognition Program Model.* Retrieved May 14, 2014. http://www.nursecredentialing.org/magnet/programoverview/new-magnet-model

Boden, D. 1994. *The Business of Talk: organizations in action.* Cambridge, England: Polity Press.

Casida, J. and J. Parker. 2011. Staff nurse perceptions of nurse manager leadership styles and outcomes. *Journal of Nursing Management 19*, 478–486.

Cherry, K. 2014. *Leadership Theories: The 8 Major Leadership Theories.* Retrieved May 17, 2014.http://www.work911.com/cgi-bin/leadership/jump.cgi?ID=10594

Cummings, G.G., T. MacGregregor, M. Davey, H. Lee, C.A. Wong., E. LO, M. Muise, and E. Stafford. 2008. *Leadership styles and outcome patterns for nursing workforce environment: A systemic review.*

Curtis, E.A., J. de Vires, and F.K. Sheerin. 2011. Developing leadership in nursing: exploring core factors. *British Journal of Nursing 20*, 5, 306–309.

Daft, R.L. and P.G. Lane. 2008. *The leadership experience 5th ed.* Mason, OH: South-Western Cengage Learning.

Fawcett, J. and J. Garity. 2009. *Evaluating Research for Evidenced-Based Nursing Practice.* F.A. Davis: Philadelphia, PA.

Freshwater, D. and T. Stickley. "The Heart of the Art: Emotional Intelligence and Nursing Education," *Nursing Inquiry,* Vol. 11, No. 2, 2004, pp. 91–98.

Guyton, N. 2012. Nine principles of successful nursing leadership. *American Nurse Today* (7), 8, retrieved May 17, 2014. http://www.americannursetoday.com/article.aspx?id=9372&fid=9326

Interprofessional Education Collaborative Expert Panel. 2011. Core competencies for interprofessional collaborative practice: Report of an expert panel. Washington, D.C.: Interprofessional Education Collaborative.

Marquis, B.L. and C.J. Huston. 2009. *Leadership Roles and Management Functions in Nursing: Theory and Application.* Philadelphia PA: Wolters Kluwer/ Lippincott.

Mayer, J.D., P. Salovey, and D. Caruso. Models of Emotional Intelligence, 2nd ed., In: Sternberg, R.J. Ed., *Handbook of Intelligence*, Cambridge, New York, 2000, pp. 396–420.

Reed, M. and B. Winston. 2005. Towards a deeper understanding of hope and leadership. *Journal of Leadership and Organizational Studies, 12*(2), 42–53.

Sullivan, E.J. and G. Garland. 2010. *Practical Leadership and Management in Nursing.* Pearson Education Limited; Harlow.

Spector, P.E. 2006. *Industrial and Organizational Psychology: Research and Practice. 4th ed.* John Wiley & Sons: New Jersey.

Stanley, D. 2006a. In command of care: Toward the theory of congruent leadership. *Journal of Nursing Research 11*(2), 132–144.

Stanley, D. 2006b. Recognizing and defining clinical nurse leaders. *British Journal of Nursing 15* (2), 108–111.

Taylor, R. 2009. Leadership theories and the development of nurses in primary health care. *Primary Health Care. 19*(9), 40–45.

Weihrich, H. and H. Koontz. 2005. *Management a Global Perspective. 11th ed.*, McGraw Hill, Singapore.

Winston, B.E. and K. Patterson. 2006. An Integrative Definition of Leadership. *International Journal of Leadership Studies 1*, 2, pp. 6–66.

Understanding Leadership, Change, and the Role of Nurse Practitioners in Clinical Practice Settings

DENISE M. KORNIEWICZ PHD., RN, FAAN

The Chapter 2 case study highlights several leadership and change theories associated with the application of these concepts for nurse practitioners working in healthcare organizations.

Case Presentation

Nancy Transman DNP is a primary care nurse practitioner in Transit, North Carolina. For over 8 years, Nancy has worked with Dr. James Bergman, a family practice physician. When Nancy began with Dr. Bergman he was in a solo practice, however within the last month his practice was purchased by the Rural Primary Care Practice System of Eastern North Carolina (RPCSENC). As a result, the practice site was moved, computerized, and accrued a large patient load and additional staff hired by RPCSENC.

The new practice team now consisted of Dr. Bergman and two other family practice physicians, four new nurse practitioners, two RNs, five medical assistants, two secretaries, and an office manager. Dr. Bergman was named as the chief medical officer at the practice site and Nancy was appointed as the supervisor over all professional and paraprofessional staff since she was the most experienced.

Nancy's only management experience consisted of being a head nurse on a step-down unit. She had not been in the role of a manager for over 5 years since she became APN. She was asked to take on these added functions with a reduced workload: 20% of her time would be freed up to manage other personnel in the practice. Her new functions would include coordinating the schedule for all staff, evaluating their job performance, and maintaining the appropriate licensures and paperwork needed to remain in compliance with RPCPSENC.

During the first month of her new position, Nancy had one meeting with all personnel and told them about the new rules and policies associated with RPCSENC. She let the staff know that she would be monitoring their performance and would meet with them as needed. At the end of the meeting several staff members approached her and stated that they did not appreciate being told that she would be monitoring their performance.

As the members of the practice began to use the new computerized programs for patient care and as more and more patients began to use their services, Dr. Bergman noticed that staff were quitting at a 35% higher rate than in the past. Everyone in the organization respected Dr. Bergman because he was charismatic, motivated, and emphasized the importance of everyone's work. Dr. Bergman spoke with Nancy about alternate ways that she could interact with other staff members so that they felt that they were valued.

As Nancy began to adjust to a larger practice and her increased responsibilities, she began to understand that how she acted or reacted impacted other team members. After being in the position for over 9 months, her staff meetings became more and more interactive and people began to be more cooperative. Additionally, she noted that staff were more involved with their work and depended on her feedback related to quality patient care.

One year later, Nancy and Dr. Bergman were notified by RPCSENC that they were being sold to a new primary care health service known as Primary Care Team Associates (PCTA). Nancy was informed that she had to prepare the staff for major changes within the organization including changes in the electronic medical records (EMR); job responsibilities, descriptions, and functions; and several internal and external processes related to patient referrals. The complexity of these changes within the healthcare system would require the primary care providers to adapt quickly to the organizational changes required by PCTA.

As a result, Nancy embarked on building a small team of primary care providers who would learn the new EMR system as well as the policies and procedures required by PCTA. She provided support services for this group and identified them as the "advocate team." The advocate team members were given the opportunity to learn the systems daily, with reduced workload related to their other functions. Once they were proficient, they were given the opportunity to teach the other primary care providers. Within one month, over 90% of the primary care staff were using the new systems and had adjusted to the organizational requirements of PCTA.

Nancy understood that being a leader required additional management skills. Because of her previous management skills she readily adapted to the organizational changes required by PCTA and was able to encourage others with the change processes. As a result, Nancy communicated with the other administrators within PCTA and suggested other change strategies that would be successful.

ESSENTIAL LEADERSHIP SKILLS FOR ADVANCE PRACTICE NURSES

Today's healthcare system is rapidly changing. With the development of the Healthcare Affordability Act (Gruber 2010), more and more individuals will seek primary care services and have 24-hour access to a primary care provider. APNs will continue to be in high demand in both primary and acute care settings. Not only is the number of APNs increasing but also the overall structure of the healthcare system is in a state of constant flux. The changes in the way healthcare systems are being reimbursed is directly tied to value or performance based reimbursement.

Nancy Transman DNP is a primary care nurse practitioner in Transit, North Carolina. For over 8 years, Nancy has worked with Dr. James Bergman, a family practice physician. When Nancy began with Dr. Bergman he was in a solo practice, however within the last month his practice was purchased the Rural Primary Care Practice System of Eastern North Carolina (RPCSENC). As a result, the practice site was moved, computerized, and accrued a large patient load and additional staff hired by RPCSENC.

The new practice team now consisted of Dr. Bergman and two other family practice physicians, four new nurse practitioners, two RNs, five medical assistants, two secretaries, and an office manager. Dr. Bergman was named as the chief medical officer at the practice site and Nancy was appointed as the supervisor over all professional and paraprofessional staff since she was the most experienced.

A variety of computerized management systems are being utilized to develop, monitor, and enhance clinical guidelines that directly impact the quality of care provided. These structural and regulatory changes have a direct impact on the leadership skills necessary to survive in healthcare environments such as independent or group practices or being part of a larger healthcare system. The need to manage individual or populations of patients demands a variety of clinical management skills that are different from today. For example, comprehensive leadership and management clinical theories used in large health systems are reflective of the mission and goals of the organization and are directly tied to the number of patients hospitalized, medical diagnosis, and specialty medical practices. Clinical theories associated with the everyday management of individual patients are leadership skills associated with the personal characteristics of an independent healthcare provider or the APN. Thus, APNs who enter the current healthcare system may need to develop an understanding of leadership or management skills that can be readily adapted within any clinical environment.

Often the development of clinical leadership theories have been applied from the principles of economics or business models that perpetuate accounting principles. Because healthcare systems are large corporations dependent on an economical model that demands productive accountable benchmarks, health professionals have been educated contrary to those principles. Most healthcare professionals such as have been exposed to noneconomic models that support concepts associated with caring, healing, or the more humanitarian approaches consistent with values perpetuated by a practiced discipline. Thus, the type of leadership used within a healthcare organization may be dependent on the expected behaviors that best describe the organization.

> Nancy's only management experience consisted of being a head nurse on a step-down unit. She had not been in the role of a manager for over 5 years since she became an APN. She was asked to take on these added functions with a reduced workload: 20% of her time would be freed up to manage other personnel in the practice. Her new functions would include coordinating the schedule for all staff, evaluating their job performance, and maintaining the appropriate licensures and paperwork needed to remain in compliance with RPCPSENC.

Historically, as healthcare organizations emerged and as social scientists began to assess organizational behavior, a cadre of leadership theories were developed. These theories ranged from descriptors associated with the characteristics of individual leadership styles to more complex systematic analyses of the interactions between leaders, workers, and the environment (Kotter and Schlesinger 2008). For example, post-World War II, leadership styles were directly related to an individual trait and described as autocratic, democratic, or laissez-fair.

During the first month of her new position, Nancy had one meeting with all personnel and told them about the new rules and policies associated with RPCSENC. She let the staff know that she would be monitoring their performance and would meet with them as needed. At the end of the meeting several staff members approached her and stated that they did not appreciate being told that she would be monitoring their performance.

However, as leadership theories continued to develop, more emphasis was placed on the leader's understanding of how his leadership style impacted workers as well as the worker's interaction with others in the work environment. For example, today the styles of leadership have been expanded to include transformational, transactional, and authentic (Table 2.1).

TABLE 2.1. Characteristics of Leadership Styles.

Leadership Style	Description and Characteristics
Autocratic	Top down approach, strong control over groups. Others are motivated by coercion or directed by command. Communication flows downward in organization and decisions do not involve others. Criticism of this style is punitive and does not support creativity.
Democratic	Less control over situations, motivational rewards are used, others are guided and communication flows up and down the organization. Decisions involve others and criticism is constructive.
Laissez-fair	Little control and no direction are provided over others. Group's complete communication flows up and down, decision-making and no criticism is used to improve organization.
Transformational	Visionary leaders motivate. Communication is up and down by sharing information and shared leadership. Criticism is discussed and shared for improvements within the organization.
Transactional	Nonvisionary leaders follow procedures and policies consistent with the organization. Often solutions are top down, and innovation or creativity is minimal.
Authentic	Visionary, charismatic leaders with great self-awareness. Communication is shared throughout the organization and teams are built to develop others. Authentic leaders provide trust and empower others in the organization.

PRINCIPLES OF LEADERSHIP FOR APNs IN HEALTHCARE ORGANIZATIONS

The role of the APN has evolved within many healthcare organizations as the demand for primary care services has increased, as legislation that defines and supports the role of the APN has changed, and as consumers have accepted patient care services rendered by APNs. Historically, the role of the APN was based in rural settings where access to healthcare services was limited. However, today APNs work in a variety of healthcare settings such as group family practice centers, specialty practice services such as internal medicine or cardiology, or within large healthcare systems that provide follow up services to specific patient populations. It is interesting to note that, from an organizational perspective, the role of an APN has been accepted in both primary and acute care settings. However, the leadership characteristics of the APN's role regardless of the healthcare setting requires autonomy, clarity of job description, and accountability (Bothma *et al.* 2011).

APNs have had to become skilled in understanding their own leadership abilities and how they influence the outcomes of patient care. Often the healthcare system and the indirect interaction among other health professionals has placed increased leadership demands on APNs. For example, most APNs have had to adjust to working within a clinical environment that provides direct patient care services within a larger system. As a result of their job function, they may be involved with transforming the healthcare system either directly or indirectly. Thus, an understanding of leadership styles consistent with organizational change is needed.

> As the members of the practice began to use the new computerized programs for patient care and as more and more patients began to use their services, Dr. Bergman noticed that staff were quitting at a 35% higher rate than in the past. Everyone in the organization respected Dr. Bergman because he was charismatic, motivated, and emphasized the importance of everyone's work. Dr. Bergman spoke with Nancy about some ways that she could interact with other staff members so that they felt that they were valued.

Transformational versus Transactional Leadership

Transformational leaders have been defined as individuals who are charismatic or visionary. They inspire and motivate others and work well in supervisory relationships such as the interaction of the supervisor and supervisee role. For the APN, this close relationship may be between the patient and APN, or the APN may be viewed as a "first level leader" within the healthcare organization because of his functional abilities. Transformational leaders assist major organizations by reinforcing the goals of the leader. Transformational APN leaders assist in multidisciplinary team building by changing attitudes, values, and behaviors while emphasizing the shared vision of the leader. One example of an APN who was a transformational leader is Loretta Ford since she transformed the nursing profession by initiating a movement that changed the delivery of healthcare so much that the word "nurse practitioner" is nearly synonymous with the name "Loretta Ford" (Giltinane 2013).

Transactional leaders are individuals who have contemporary management styles consistent with monitoring performance and interceding with corrective action when necessary. Transactional leaders often are nonvisionary and employ management techniques that implicate policy or procedure versus cultural change. Often, transactional leaders are described as reactive and supportive of the "status quo" (Avolio *et al.* 2009). Transactional leaders can offer prompt solutions to problems for immediate staff needs especially during times of stress or crisis. Depending on the role of the APN within a healthcare organization, this style of leadership may be necessary when trying to implement a new policy or demonstrate specific patient care outcomes. Thus, a transactional leadership style may be appropriate in many clinical settings, but not necessarily open to innovation.

As Nancy began to adjust to a larger practice and her increased responsibilities, she began to understand that how she acted or reacted impacted other team members. After being in the position for over 9 months, her staff meetings became more and more interactive and people began to be more cooperative. Additionally, she noted that staff were more involved with their work and depended on her feedback related to quality patient care.

Authentic Leadership

Authentic leadership has been defined as a process that incorporates the positive psychological capacities of an individual and the promotion of greater self-awareness, self-regulation, and positive behaviors of a leader (Avolio and Gardner 2005). Shamir and Eilam (2005) suggested four general characteristics associated with authentic leadership styles. These include: (1) true-to-self versus conforming to the expectations of others, (2) motivations are personal convictions versus personal benefits, (3) leadership is original versus from a personal point of view, and (4) a leadership style is based on personal values and convictions. Authentic leaders are confident, optimistic, hopeful, and resilient. They are able to motivate and involve their followers to constantly improve their work and continue to strive for excellent performance outcomes. Authentic leaders act on their beliefs by being the person they are and consistently demonstrate behaviors such as speaking the truth, leading from the heart, having strong morals, being courageous, building teams, understanding themselves, committing to excellence, and leaving a legacy by developing others.

Wong *et al.* (2010) demonstrated that authentic leaders were able to influence other healthcare providers by enabling trust in the manager and engaging professionals to work in one direction, thus impacting the overall quality of patient care provided. This leadership style has a significant impact in clinical environments by providing positive direction for work group engagement to increase positive patient outcomes and in sustaining healthy work environments. Thus, APNs who foster a trusting work environment without reprisal from multidisciplinary staff members would directly impact the quality of patient care and provide functional healthy workplaces.

The use of the authentic leadership style in clinical practice settings provides a positive way to develop the skills necessary to successfully navigate complex healthcare systems. Application of the attributes related to authentic leadership to APN practice may be directly associated with the APNs relationship with the patient. For example, patients who trust their primary care provider or APN are more apt to foster self-care health outcomes such as medication compliance or the practice of healthy life style behaviors. APNs who apply these leadership characteristics to the management of healthcare team members within a clinical practice may increase the overall performance of quality patient care rendered by clinical staff.

One year later, Nancy and Dr. Bergman were notified by RPC-SENC that they were being sold to a new primary care health service known as Primary Care Team Associates (PCTA). Nancy was informed that she had to prepare the staff for major changes within the organization including changes in the electronic medical records (EMR); job responsibilities, descriptions, and functions; and several internal and external processes related to patient referrals. The complexity of these changes within the healthcare system would require the primary care providers to adapt quickly to the organizational changes required by PCTA.

THEORIES OF CHANGE

Today, APNs continue to work in a changing healthcare atmosphere which requires constant adaptation, and the ability to build relationships with interdisciplinary healthcare teams and to survive in a complex multilevel organization. The skills required to positively influence and motivate members of a working team require an understanding of a variety of change theories that impact their ability to be successful.

There are several theories that have been used to explain change within any large healthcare system. The general concepts that are used to explain the change process usually describe the interactions of the change agent with the internal and external environment. Depending on one's role in the change process, interaction of the change agent within the healthcare system is dependent on three barriers: self, the target environment, and the external environment. For example, Kurt Lewin's theory of change (1947) describes three phases that occur during a change process: periods of unfreezing, periods of moving, and periods of refreezing. For several years, healthcare leaders applied Lewin's theory of change to explain or analyze why a change process either worked or did not work within the healthcare environment. However, as healthcare systems became more complicated and complex, a variety of organizational theories were developed to understand the change process, the principles of leadership, and the process of human behavior associated with change. Today, the most common change theories include complexity theory, Kotter's eight-step process for change, and the principles of innovation and change.

Complexity Science and Change

Complexity science is an organizational framework that explores the role of organizational leadership and the process of how individuals adapt to change within an organization, and investigates how members of the organization begin to govern themselves through self-regulation and adaptation (Martin and Sturmberg 2005). APNs working in these complex health systems often have to work within professional groups, departments, or specialties that require nonlinear interactions within the groups. This may result in communication patterns that conflict with each other versus efficient or constructive organizational supports. Nurse practitioners who adapt to the demands of their environment, such as understanding how their behavior impacts the work environment, often emerge as clinical leaders who provide the organizational structures that enhance quality patient care. Thus, change results from the interaction of the system members as they adapt to new situations, and leadership emerges at all levels within the organization.

The application of complexity science to the role of the nurse practitioner is specifically related to how APNs interact with the clinical
environment. Since this requires individuals to adapt to both the physical and psychological changes within the work environment, APNs
cannot force patients to adapt to their own health situation. Rather,
APNs need to use this leadership style when working with patients
so that the patients can tackle their own health problems (Bailey *et
al.* 2012). For example, at the point of care, APNs can use an "adaptive
leadership" style to assist patients to make behavior changes of self-
regulation and to have control over their own health. Patients would
have to re-evaluate their existing beliefs and learn to adopt new priorities and habits related to their own health. These change processes
engage patients in the self-management of their chronic illness and
provide an organizational structure of adapting, learning, and making
behavioral changes.

Kotter's Eight-Stage Change Process

Kotter (1996) outlined an eight-step process for leading change
within an organization. These eight principles provide a systematic framework to successfully create change within an organization. Nurse practitioners who work in complex health systems may
be asked to initiate a change process that requires a systematic approach and encompasses all healthcare providers. One example may
be the initiation of a new EMR computer system that requires patient
centered initiatives. In order to fulfill a task of this nature, the APNs
would need an understanding of a change process. Embedded in Kotter's (2001) eight-step process are the following organizational steps:
(1) establish an urgency, (2) create a coalition, (3) develop a vision,
(4) communicate the vision, (5) empower others, (6) generate wins, (7)
never let up, and (8) incorporate cultural change. In order to be successful at increasing healthcare worker compliance in using the EMR
within the clinical setting, the APNs would set goals for each of the
steps within the change process (Table 2.2).

Others (Gruber and Jonathan 2010; Frankel *et al.* 2006) have demonstrated that the use of these guiding principles have assisted in successfully changing the culture of the organization. Therefore, the APNs
may be involved in leading changes within a clinical environment and
providing feedback to others as the change is implemented.

APNs can use these same steps to lead change processes when working with individual patients or with groups of patients. Using Kotter's
(2001) model to initiate step one, the APNs working with a noncompliant diabetic patient would create a sense of urgency about the patient's

TABLE 2.2. Kotter's Eight-step process for Leading Change as Applied to Organizations and Patients.

Change Step Definition	Application Within a Healthcare System	Application with Patient
1. Establish a sense of urgency	Help other healthcare professionals see what needs to be changed or improved.	Empower patient to perceive health need.
2. Create coalitions of support	Build teams that will encourage change processes.	Build family/significant other support structures to help the patient make changes in health behavior.
3. Develop a vision to change	Preplan change effort among constituents by developing strategies for change.	Work with family members to plan successful change strategies for patient.
4. Communicate the vision for buy-in	Talk to as many people as possible within the organization to facilitate an understanding of what the change is; explore alternate strategies for communication.	Talk to extended family or significant friends of patient to facilitate an understanding of the changes needed for patient's health status.
5. Empower broad-based action	Remove any obstacles to the change process or structures that would undermine the process. May include changing personnel, policies, or organizational structures.	Strategize with family and significant others to be sure to remove the patient's family members that are not supportive of change. Institute group support systems so patient can feel empowered.
6. Generate short term wins	Acknowledge achievements that can be made visible to others in the organization and reward employees involved in the changes process.	Acknowledge positive outcomes through rewards to patient for changing behavior such as providing a reward or patient newsletter acknowledgement.
7. Never let up	Provide changes in the structures or policies that support the change or vision by promoting or hiring employees that support the new changes.	Provide treatment changes consistent with attained goals. Demonstrate to patient impact on their own health needs through feedback and positive communication.
8. Incorporate changes into the culture	Articulate all organizational changes resulting from successes by employees. Ensure leadership development and succession.	Provide positive feedback to patient and provide ways that will ensure behavioral changes. This may include the development of patients as coaches to other patients so they can assist in the change process.

blood glucose levels. The APNs would provide a variety of techniques to educate the patient about the consequences associated with noncompliance through educational videos that show adverse health effects related to cardiovascular strokes, amputations, or kidney failure. The APNs would provide opportunities for further follow up and discussions with the patient so that overtime, the patient positively encompasses the change process.

> As a result, Nancy embarked on building a small team of primary care providers who would learn the new EMR system as well as the policies and procedures required by PCTA. She provided support services for this group and identified them as the "advocate team." The advocate team members were given the opportunity to learn the systems daily, with reduced workload related to their other functions. Once they were proficient, they were given the opportunity to teach the other primary care providers. Within one month, over 90% of the primary care staff were using the new systems and had adjusted to the organizational requirements of PCTA.

Diffusion of Innovation and Change

Innovation has been defined as a process that occurs when an idea is introduced and when members of the organization use it. In healthcare organizations, Berwick (2008) suggested that healthcare workers needed to be competent at using a new product or innovation before adapting it to their environment. The fusion of innovation research has attempted to explain the concepts associated with how and why users adapt to change or new information. Rogers (1995) described innovation as a four-stage process consisting of: (1) invention, (2) diffusion (or communication) through the social system, (3) time, and (4) consequences. Application of Rogers' theory to the healthcare environment would include studying the behavior of healthcare workers involved in a change process or the use of a new product. Further, the fusion of the innovation change process has been described as having five sub-categories in to which individuals "fit" as they adopt to change, including: (1) innovators, (2) early adopters, (3) early majority, (4) late majority, and (5) laggards (Table 2.3).

Within each of these categories, the message is communicated over time and individuals begin to adapt to the new idea and communicate to others or share information with one another to reach a mutual understanding (Doran *et al.* 2010).

Application of innovation and change among APNs may be viewed in

TABLE 2.3. *Change Theory: Diffusion of Innovation and Description.*

Change Adopters	Description
Innovators	Individuals who are the first to take risk and adopt an innovation or new technology.
Early adopters	Individuals who are opinionated and adopt an innovation or technology because they are discrete and do not want to maintain the "status quo."
Early Majority	Individuals who adopt an innovation after a period of time. Usually, the adoption period is significantly longer than the innovators than early adopters. Early Majority adopters tend to be slower in the adoption process.
Late Majority	These individuals approach an innovation with a high degree of skepticism and after the majority of people have adopted the innovation they will adopt it.
Laggards	Last group of individuals to adopt an innovation or new technology. Laggards are described as individuals who are focused on "traditions" and will not adopt until family or friends adopt.

two ways. First, from an organizational systems perspective where adaptation of a new computer-tracking program has been initiated. APNs working within a primary care practice would support the program to increase the quality of patient care standards and the need to standardize treatment options. The process from initiation to adaptation would be tracked to provide feedback associated with the percent of individuals who assisted in the innovation to use the new computer program. General data would be provided to assess the percent of early adopters to the program and comparisons would be made as to why others adopted at later times. By communicating the outcomes associated with the change process and providing time to use the new product, primary care providers would understand and institute the changes needed.

A second application of innovation and change can be by individual APNs who provide primary care services to patient populations. For example, a change process may include the use of cell phones among patients to encourage self-care and behavior change related to treatment or prevention. The process would include teaching the patient to use the software application on his cell phone and direct feedback from the primary provider would be given. Again, feedback to the patient or group of patients would be provided and the APNs could rate the numbers of early and late adaptors who use this new technology. Therefore, the fusion of innovation and change can be readily adapted to major organizations, minor subsystems such as group practices, or to patient populations.

FUTURE ROLE OF APNs IN HEALTHCARE ORGANIZATIONS

As a result of the Healthcare Affordability Act, it is estimated that 32 million more Americans will require primary care services (Gruber and Jonathan 2010). Further, the Association of American Medical Colleges estimates that by 2015 that there will be a shortage of 33,000 family practice physicians (Berwick *et al.* 2008). Due to the regulation of re-imbursement patterns, legislative mandates associated with the "scope of practice" for APNs, and issues related to access to care, the role of the APNs will continue to be needed. Thus, the skills associated with effective leadership, an understanding of healthcare organizations, and the ability to understand safe practices and accountability measures are paramount to the success of the APNs role.

Nancy understood that being a leader required additional manage-ment skills. Because of her previous management skills she readily adapted to the organizational changes required by PCTA and was able to encourage others with the change processes. As a result, Nan-cy communicated with the other administrators within PCTA and suggested other change strategies that would be successful.

APNs will continue to be primary care providers as the demand for pri-mary care services increase. Perhaps there will be some expansion of the role of the APNs as healthcare systems continue to reorganize and provide cost-effective health options. For example, in some specialty services such as oncology, surgery, and cardiac, APNs work with physician specialists by providing discharge and follow-up to specific patient populations. A second expanded role for the APNs will be the need to provide out-patient services that are convenient for patients, such as APNs working in conjunc-tion with pharmacists, and being available when patients have questions associated with their treatments. Additionally, several outpatient facilities may be open 24 hours and APNs will become the primary care provider. Third, APNs will continue to be the primary care providers in urban and rural underserved areas since most physician providers refuse to work in those areas. Last, the need for APNs may be expanded into academia since the academic workforce is aging and the need to provide competent clini-cal experts to educate future APNs will become more of a necessity.

SUMMARY POINTS

- APNs need to apply leadership principles to be effective primary care providers.

- The role of APNs requires an understanding of transformation, transactional, and authentic leadership styles to provide quality patient care.
- An APN's knowledge about his own behavior influences others in the clinical environment and impacts the overall performance of exceptional patient care.
- An understanding of change theories, including complexity science, Kotter's eight-stage change process, and the theory of innovation, is essential knowledge for APNs.
- The application of a change process is necessary when working in a healthcare system or when working with individuals or groups of patients.

REFERENCES

Avolio, B.J. and W. Gardner. 2005. Authentic leadership development: Getting to the root of positive forms of leadership. *The Leadership Quarterly 16*, 315–338.

Avolio, B.J., F.O. Walumbwa, and T.J. Weber. 2009. Leadership:current theories, research, and future directions. *Annual Review of Psychology 60*, 421–449.

Bailey, D., S.L. Docherty, J.A. Adams, *et al.* 2012. Studying the clinical encounter with the adaptive leadership framework. *Journal of Healthcare Leadership 4*,83–91.

Berwick, D., T. Nolao, and J. Whittingtton. 2008. The triple aim: care, health, and cost. *Health Affairs 27*, no. 3 (2008): 759–769.

Botma, Y., H. Botha, and M. Nel. 2011. Transformation: are nurse leaders in critical care ready? *Journal of Nursing Management, 20*, 921–927.

Doran, D.M., B. Haynes, and A. Kusniruk, *et al.* 2010. Supporting evidence-based practice for nurses through information technologies. *Worldviews on Evidence-Based Nursing; 7*(1):4–15

Frankel, A., M. Leonard, and C. Denham. 2006. Fair and Just Culture, Team Behavior, and Leadership Engagement: The Tools to Achieve High Reliability. *Health Serv Res.* 2006 August; 41(4 Pt 2): 1690–1709.

Giltinane, C.L. 2013. Leadership styles and theories. *Nursing Standard. 27*, 41, 35–39.

Gruber, J. 2010. The Cost Implications of Health Care Reform. *New England Journal of Medicine 362* (22), 2050–2051.

Kotter, J. 1996. *Leading Change.* Harvard business school press.

Kotter, J. 2001. What leaders really do. *Harvard business review, 12*, 3–11.

Kotter, J. and L. Schlesinger. 2008. Choosing strategies for change. *Harvard business review, 7*, 1–11.

Lewin, K. 1947. Frontiers in group dynamics, in: D. Cartwright (Ed.) (1952): *Field Theory in social Science.* Social Science Paperbacks: London.

Martin, C.M. and J.P. Sturmberg. 2005. General practice—chaos, complexity and innovation. *MJA, 183*, 2, 106–109.

Rogers, E.M. 1995. *Diffusion of Innovations.* 5th ed. New York, NY: Free Press.

Shamir, B. and G. Eilam. 2005. What's your story A life-stories approach to authentic leadership development. *The Leadership Quarterly.*

Wong, C., H. Lashinger, and G. Cummings. 2010. Authentic leadership and nurses' voice behaviour and perceptions of care quality. *Journal of Nursing Management, 2010, 18,* 889–900.

Safe Leadership Practices

DENISE M. KORNIEWICZ PHD., RN, FAAN
JEANNE H. SIEGEL PHD., ARNP

The Chapter 3 case study explores the legal issues associated with leadership decisions that impact safe, clinical decision making for advanced practice professionals.

Case Presentation

Dr. Marilyn Sprague DNP, ARNP, BC recently relocated to south Florida and landed the job of Vice President (VP) of Nursing at a well-known, large medical system which consisted of six regional hospitals and one main hospital. The hospitals were purchased over the previous 6 years and had their own leadership structures. Until the appointment of a system-wide VP of Nursing, each hospital nursing staff had made its own policy and procedure decisions. The director of nursing (DON) at each institution made all of the hiring and termination decisions. There were no system-wide policies and procedures, committees, or approval processes, and review of these documents were sporadic and disorganized.

The president of the medical system made the decision to recruit a system VP of Nursing since there were several concerns related to poor patient outcomes. Two of the regional hospitals had serious citations from the Joint Commission on Accreditation of Healthcare Organizations (JCAHO) and one of the magnet hospitals had not been renewed due to failure to provide leadership for a safe clinical practice environment. The major safe practice issue was an increase in hospital acquired (nosocomial) infections across the hospital.

Marilyn knew she had a tough job ahead in developing a system-wide leadership structure, committees, policies and procedures, and effective risk management and compliance mechanisms. One of her major concerns was the potential liability the system faced, not only from malpractice exposure, but also fines and penalties for failure to meet the requirements of government and certifying body regulations. There was no system-wide tracking and reporting of patient injury (falls, infection, surgical complications, and deaths). The hospitals that had risk managers did not have clear reporting requirements or policies and procedures. Further investigation found that the nurse leadership from the regional hospitals never met on a regular basis and there was no formal meeting or communication structure between them.

The system did not have a centralized "risk management" department and tracking of all risk management statistics and incident reporting was performed at the individual hospitals. As a consequence, there was no ability to gather system-wide statistical data or to make meaningful comparisons on patient outcomes.

The main hospital did have one in-house attorney who was tasked with overseeing legal issues for the entire system. But when asked about his role, the attorney stated, "I rarely get calls from the regional facilities. I am here if they need me."

Marilyn was also in charge of researching and making recommendations for a system-wide electronic health record (EHR) and a documentation/communication system that met Health Information Portability and Accountability Act of 1997 (HIPAA) and other governmental regulatory requirements. This system was to be a functional unit that was to be used throughout the system and nursing needs were to be the first to implement it.

Current research at the hospitals appeared to be based out of the local medical school. Consequently, research protocols created unnecessary conflict with the hospitals operations. There was an IRB for the main hospital, but nursing representation was absent. However, not one of the hospital policy or procedure committees used an evidence-based practice model. As a result, Marilyn knew that she had to begin to develop a system-wide approach to monitoring patient care practices.

ESSENTIAL LEGAL CONCERNS FOR APNs

Advance practice nursing requires individuals to understand the issues related to safe clinical practice from the perspectives of clinical accountability and professional leadership. Depending on the role of the APN within the healthcare system, issues such as licensure, certification, credentialing, patient's rights, negligence, and malpractice impact leadership decisions and safe patient care. Within the microsystem of APNs providing direct patient care, clinical leadership involves promoting changes that directly impact patient outcomes, clinical guideline development, and the promotion of evidence-based clinical standards. Professional leadership expands the role of the APN as a leader who influences healthcare reform by contributing to the development of policies that help shape the delivery of healthcare (Begley *et al.* 2012). Regardless of what role the APN may be employed, an understanding of safe leadership practices that may have legal implications is essential.

> Dr. Marilyn Sprague DNP, APN, BC recently relocated to south Florida and landed the job of VP of Nursing at a well-known large medical system which consisted of six regional hospitals and one main hospital. The hospitals were purchased over the previous 6 years and had their own leadership structures. Until the appointment of a system-wide VP of Nursing, each hospital nursing staff had made its own policy and procedure decisions. The DON at each institution made all of the hiring and termination decisions. There were no system-wide policies and procedures, committees, or approval processes and review of these documents were sporadic and disorganized.

The primary purposes of the laws applicable to healthcare are to protect the interests of the patient. APNs will encounter issues associated with licensure, certification, informed consent, medical records, and confidentiality. Being aware of the relevant federal and state laws and regulations can help protect the patient, practitioner, and the healthcare facility.

Licensure and Certification

Because APNs work in healthcare systems at a variety of levels, it is imperative that the overall health system provides a uniform organizational matrix that provides oversight for licensure, certification, and credentialing. Licensure merely is the ability of a governing agency that grants permission to obtain a license to provide health services to patients. Obtaining a license provides assurance to the public that minimum qualifications have been met to provide healthcare to individuals, families, or communities.

The APN consensus model (NCSBN 2008) defined the role of advanced practice registered nurses to include certified nurse midwives, certified nurse practitioners, certified nurse anesthetists, and certified clinical nurse specialists. As a result, all APNs must be initially licensed as a registered nurse and then certified as an advanced practice registered nurse (APRN). Certification and use of the legal title APRN requires that individuals have graduated from an accredited APRN educational program, are nationally certified, and are licensed under the criteria delineated in the APRN consensus model (NCSBN 2008). All graduates of APRN programs must be able to pass a national certification exam that assures competent and advanced safe clinical practice. The use of a uniform title and credentialing of the APRN will allow easy recognition by the public, policy makers, and other health professionals. The target date to incorporate the use of APRN throughout the United States is 2015, thus new legislation will need to be drafted in states that do not currently use the APRN legal title. Use of this title is not restricted by setting but is patient-centered and provides enhanced scope of practice for APNs (Stanley, 2012).

The President of the Medical System made the decision to recruit a system VP of Nursing since there were several concerns related to poor patient outcomes. Two of the regional hospitals had serious citations from the Joint Commission on Accreditation of Healthcare Organizations (JCAHO) and one of the magnet hospitals had not been renewed due to failure to provide leadership for a safe clinical practice environment. The major safe practice issue was an increase in hospital acquired (nosocomial) infections across the hospital.

Patient Rights/Informed Consent

In 1995, the National Health Council adopted general principles associated with a patient's rights. These included the patient's right to be informed about treatment concerns, timeliness, the ability to understand, the right to know about insurance coverage, cost of care, choice of providers, and the right to know what incentives or restrictions the provider may have when rendering care. The principles associated with the rights of patients provide a mutual framework for the patient and the healthcare provider.

In a mutually respectful relationship, shared decision-making is fundamental. In healthcare, the parties involved (provider and patient) demonstrate this relationship by using informed consent. The purpose of informed consent is to protect the patients' legal right to participate in the decisions made about their care with full disclosure of information on risks, benefits, and alternatives of a proposed treatment or surgery (Menendez 2013). The informed consent process has historically been the sole responsibility of the physician, however, today the responsibility may be with an advanced practice provider or staff within the healthcare facility. What is important is that the informed consent process is followed according to the policies or procedures outlined within the healthcare system.

Ideally, the informed consent process is seamless; the physician or other healthcare provider explains in detail the risks, benefits, and alternatives of planned procedures, treatments, or surgeries. Often, nurses are patient advocates and are instrumental in addressing issues that arise from the consenting process. Some of the situations that may occur during the consenting process may include language barriers, level of education, patient anxiety, patient's inability to understand, and refusal to consent. As a result, APNs need to be aware of the exceptions to the health system's process for obtaining a standard informed consent.

Marilyn knew she had a tough job ahead in developing a system-wide leadership structure, committees, policies and procedures, and effective risk management and compliance mechanisms. One of her major concerns was the potential liability the system faced, not only from malpractice exposure, but also fines and penalties for failure to meet the requirements of government and certifying body regulations.

Protection of Medical Records and Information

APNs in clinical leadership roles have a responsibility to understand and monitor healthcare systems for compliance to standards and regulations that protect a patient's privacy, medical information, and healthcare records. The use of a systematic, computerized method to provide privacy for patients may include computer encryption, passwords, and data codes that protect personal information about the patient. Additionally, annual training by a continuing education compliance program for all healthcare providers who have access to the medical record is suggested. However, some of the challenges may include employees who use the healthcare facility, celebrities who are hospitalized, press inquiries, photographs, family members, or the use of social networks about a hospitalized patient. Most importantly is the establishment of consistent policies and procedures that are accessible throughout the healthcare system by authorized healthcare personnel. Access to health records, the review of health data, as well as financial information need to be available for healthcare personnel who require access to the information.

Confidentiality

APNs need to be aware of creating a trusting environment by respecting patients' privacy. Often patients disclose personal information to the healthcare provider. As a result, healthcare providers have to seek permission from patients to disclose information gained through patient-provider communication. The obligation of confidentiality prohibits the healthcare provider from disclosing information about the patients' status to others without permission. Because of the use of electronic medical records and in accordance with HIPPA, the use of private information and the protection of electronic information and computerized data must be disclosed to all patients.

The most important issue associated with confidentiality as a patient provider is whether or not the APN will put another person or group at risk or serious harm. A few questions that may assist APNs with the right decision include:

1. Will the lack of patient information put another person or group at high risk or serious harm?
2. Is the information requested important for treatment for a minor in need of healthcare?
3. Does the person who is requesting the information have medical power of attorney to obtain medical records?

When in doubt, the APN should check with their risk management advisor or review the institution's guidelines associated with patient privacy.

LEGAL HAZARDS FOR APNs AS NURSE LEADERS

Historically, physicians were the healthcare providers who were held responsible for poor outcomes and liability associated with the delivery of healthcare (Marquis and Huston 2009). As nurses gained more education and experience, they have assumed the authority, autonomy, and liability for their practice and the nurses they supervise. Nurses are challenged daily with new technology, financial constraints, staffing shortages, cultural diversity, staffing skill mix, and communication difficulties with a variety of disciplines (Curtis *et al.* 2011). Because of the role that nurses occupy in the delivery of safe clinical care, the role of leader and the possession of leadership qualities are not optional (Curtis *et al.* 2011). Most nurses arrive in advanced practice leadership roles without a comprehensive understanding of the legal perils they are likely to encounter. The lack of experience, scant training, and scarce legal resources available to support the APN can lead to unforeseen and unfortunate consequences for the nurse and the employer.

APNs as nurse leaders should be knowledgeable about the legal matters they may face in their daily practice in order to protect themselves and their employees from liability and/or the loss of professional licensure (Marquis and Huston 2009). APNs, as a result of their advanced roles, are increasingly the target for malpractice lawsuits. This leads to both an increase in medical malpractice insurance rates and the loss of employment because of the increased cost employers must absorb to provide malpractice insurance to their employees (Klutz 2004). As a consequence of their education and leadership roles, APNs as nurse leaders are required to bear the cost of increasingly expensive malpractice insurance, only to discover that it increases the likelihood of being sued. Injured parties will always seek damages from as many healthcare professionals who have malpractice resources (Marquis and Huston 2009).

One unintended consequence of the increased rates of malpractice litigation is the practice of "defensive medicine" by all healthcare providers (Klutz 2004; Tuers 2013). Defensive medical practice includes unnecessary testing and increased procedures, admissions, labs studies, medications, and therapies to reduce the provider and the institutions' liability risk (Catino 2009). As a result, defensive medicine continues to tax the healthcare system and has diverted needed healthcare resources away from patients. Emergency rooms are particularly vulnerable to medical malpractice claims due to the fast pace, lack of patient-provider relationship, and patient expectations. Thus, defensive medicine costs are significantly increased and access to healthcare resources is limited (Tuers 2013).

> The system did not have a centralized "risk management" department and tracking of all risk management statistics and incident reporting was performed at the individual hospitals. As a consequence, there was no ability to gather system-wide statistical data or to make meaningful comparisons on patient outcomes.
>
> The main hospital did have one in-house attorney who was tasked with overseeing legal issues for the entire system. But when asked about his role, the attorney stated, "I rarely get calls from the regional facilities. I am here if they need me."

Malpractice and Intentional Torts

Intentional torts are intentional actions that result in harm to the plaintiff. According to Gifis (2008), a tort is "a wrong; a private or civil wrong or injury resulting from a breach of legal duty that exists by virtue of society's expectations regarding interpersonal conduct, rather than by contract or other private relationship." The harm need not be intended, but the act must be intentional, not merely careless or reckless. Most intentional torts are also crimes. Medical battery is one potential criminal tort. In order to prove battery, the five elements of act, intent, causation (actual or proximate), touching, or harm (offensive) must exist. An example of a medical assault and battery where the assault is a threat is an APN saying to a patient, "If you don't take these medications, I will force them down your throat!" Battery is the physical touching that is against the patient's will, or operating or performing a procedure without informed consent. Thus, an APN who forces medication down the throat of a patient by physically doing the act can be charged with assault and battery.

Medical malpractice is professional negligence by "act or omission" by a healthcare provider in which the treatment provided falls below the accepted standard of care in the medical or nursing community and causes injury or death to the patient, with most cases involving medical error. An example of an APN involved in a medical malpractice case is if the APN prescribed a medication that the patient is known to be allergic to and insisted that the patient take the medication anyway. As a result, the patient may have an adverse reaction and the APN would be held liable for the incident.

Professional Negligence

Professional negligence can be defined as a careless act that breeches the usual and safe standard of care. There are five elements of negligence that have been broadly defined as professional negligence: duty, breach (usual standard of care), actual causation, proximate causation, and damages. Most intentional torts are the result of negligence and occur as a result of not adhering to the established or safe standard of medical care. An example of professional negligence for a practicing APN is the failure to obtain the standard and routine number of electrocardiographic (EKG) readings required on patients who are on routine cardiac antiarrhythmic medications. Failure to monitor a patient's cardiac status as recommended by the American College of Cardiology would be considered a breach in the standard of care and result in a charge of professional negligence.

SUMMARY POINTS

• It is important for APNs to understand safe leadership practices to avoid the legal issues that may occur resulting from unsafe medical or nursing practice.

- An understanding of the guidelines associated with licensure, certification, and scope of practice are important concepts for the APN.
- APNs as nurse leaders can serve as role models by providing and expecting nursing care that meets or exceeds accepted standards of care.
- APNs possess the leadership qualities associated with safe clinical practice and the need to understand the legal issues surrounding patient care, risk management, medical malpractice, and professional negligence.

REFERENCES

American Nurse Association (ANA). 2014. *Leadership Definition.* Retrieved June 6, 2014. http://www.nursingworld.org/MainMenuCategories/The Practice of Professional Nursing/Leadership

Begley C., N. Elliott, J. Lalor, *et al.* 2012. Differences between clinical specialist and advanced practitioner clinical practice, leadership, and research roles, responsibilities, and perceived outcomes (the SCAPE study). *Journal of Advanced Nursing 69* (6) 1323–1337.

Catino, M. 2009. Blame culture and defensive medicine. *Cognition, Technology & Work, 11;4,* 245–253.

Gifis, S.H. 2008. *Barron's Dictionary of Legal Terms, 4th ed.* Barron's; Hauppauge, NY.

Health Information and Portability Act. PPA. Accessed July 2, 2014. http://www.hhs.gov/ocr/privacy/hipaa/administrative/statute/hipaastatutepdf.pdfref

Klutz, D.L. 2004. Tort Reform: An Issue for Nurse Practitioners. *Journal of the American Academy of Nurse Practitioners 16;* 2, 70–75.

Marquis, B.L.and C.J. Huston. 2009. *Leadership Roles and Management Functions in Nursing: Theory and Application.* Philadelphia PA: Wolters Kluwer/ Lippincott.

National Council of State Boards of Nursing, APRN Advisory Council. 2008. *Consensus Model for APRN Regulation: Licensure, Accreditation, Certification & Education.* I. Coyne, A. Higgins, and C.M. Comiskey. Accessed 2014.https://www.ncsbn.org/Consensus_Model_for_APRN_Regulation_July_2008.pdf

Principles of patients' rights and responsibilities. Accessed June 16, 2014. http://www.nationalhealthcouncil.org/pages/page-content.php?pageid=66

Stanley, J. 2012. Impact of New Regulatory Standards on Advanced Practice Registered Nursing. The APRN Consensus Model and LACE. *Nurs Clin N Am 47* (2012) 241–250.

Tuers, D.M. 2013. Defensive medicine in the emergency department: increasing health care costs without increasing quality? *Nurs Adm Q* April–June 37 (2) 160–4.

Understanding Health Organizations and Systems

CHRISTINE C. HARSELL DNP, ANP-BC

The Chapter 4 case study includes concepts related to evidence-based approaches to organizing clinical care in traditional and nontraditional practice settings. Additional content includes the role of the advanced practice professional in providing organizational input into clinical practice decisions.

Case Presentation

Maya is a nurse practitioner who provides primary care in a rural community. She works in a federally qualified community health center (CHC). One of her patients is on Coumadin therapy to treat a clotting disorder. The diagnosis of the disorder involved specialists and lab work which has already cost the patient thousands of dollars. Maya has had difficulty getting the Coumadin dose regulated and her patient's INR is subtherapeutic despite 4 months of regulating the dose. Maya asks her nurse to initiate a referral to the Coumadin clinic at the closest hospital system which is 50 miles away. The patient reluctantly agrees to get a consult—although she already is concerned about the costs. Upon requesting the consult, the clinic nurse learns that in order to access the Coumadin clinic services, the patient must have a primary care provider who works within the hospital system. They will not accept a patient from "outside" the system. Maya is surprised by this new rule since she has frequently collaborated with specialists at the hospital in order to provide high quality healthcare to her patients. She makes some calls herself to see if she can explain this patient's case and perhaps get an exception. She is met with immediate resistance and is again told that her patient will need to transfer her primary care to the hospital clinic system in order to utilize the Coumadin clinic services. Maya discusses the options with her patient, who refuses to leave the CHC as her primary care home. Maya is left to manage the issue without support.

At the next CHC provider meeting, Maya brings up this issue and discovers that the other providers have had similar issues when referring for services at the hospital. The infusion center will not take patients without having a primary care provider within the system and the pain clinic is considering a similar model. The providers and the CEO decide to request a meeting with the executives of the hospital to discuss their concerns and hopefully to brainstorm options that will serve the needs of their rural community. Maya is asked to take the lead in setting up the meeting and begins to prepare.

Despite her frustrations, Maya knows that she needs to try to understand why the hospital policy exists. She applies a systems thinking approach in order to understand the complexity of the issue. She brainstorms a few ideas on her own and gathers data from patients and her colleagues. She concludes that keeping patients within the same system for all their care has some obvious cost and safety benefits including efficient use of time, streamlining care, and ensuring adequate communication and follow up. Maya also knows there are a variety of consequences related to this policy that may not be beneficial to the hospital. She gathers data from her colleagues at the CHC, as well as patient stories who have been affected by this rule. Providers are feeling frustrated by having to choose between sending their patients away and not providing the best possible care. They have already begun using other hospital services less frequently because of this matter. Every patient where this has become an issue is uninsured and cannot afford the transportation or extra money that switching to a different primary care provider would cost. Maya knows that there are other potential concerns for the hospital if they continue to enforce this policy with the CHC patients including missed appointments, unpaid balances, and the likely increase in use of emergency services. She is easily able to make a case for the potential revenue lost due to this policy. Finally, she gathers crucial evidence which supports the use of primary care providers in rural areas in order to increase access and reduce health disparities.

At the meeting, Maya takes the lead and is able to succinctly state CHC's concerns, the consequences to all parties, and to make suggestions for resolution. Because of her preparation, she is able to field questions and provide evidence-based rebuttals to any concerns. Maya also has had past experience working with members of the hospital board on various community organizational committees. She knew in advance who might be willing to adopt change and who might be more resistant. She was careful to make sure her presentation won over the early adopters.

During the meeting, Maya encourages the hospital executives to identify the various external agencies that are involved in caring for patients. She helps to articulate how these separate organizations impact the hospital as well as how hospital decisions impact them; the interdependence. Through this simple process, the executive team rethinks their position related to utilization of specialty services and their hospital and revises the policy to include patients from outlying areas and related agencies like the CHC. Maya is especially pleased when she is asked to be a part of a task force made up of stakeholders from the hospital and the interrelated external systems as they plan to expand services into other rural areas.

ESSENTIAL CONTENT FOR UNDERSTANDING ORGANIZATIONS AND SYSTEMS

As nurses continue to lead the charge in improving patient health, it has become even more important for nurse leaders to be comfortable working within health systems to assess problems, identify solutions, and make change. The American Association of Colleges of Nursing (AACN) Essentials of Doctoral Education for Advanced Nursing Practice calls for practitioners with skills in organizational and systems leadership (AACN 2006). This chapter provides an overview of organizational theories, system thinking and evaluation, patient centered care, and organizational change processes.

Organizations and Systems

An organization, simply put, is a group of individuals with specific responsibilities who are working together for a common purpose or goal. Within an organization, there is also structure and processes within which the individuals in an organization interact (Huber 2010). Organizations are mission oriented and often provide a vision or expected outcome of the individuals who support the organization.

Organizations can be viewed as open or closed systems. A closed system is a system that has little to no interaction with its outside environment. It is compartmentalized and favors defined structures and processes that are often hierarchical in nature. Leaders in closed systems conduct their work in an attempt to control the internal environment and keep minimal influence from the external environment (Greene 2005).

The functional nursing care delivery model is an example of a closed system. Nurses and staff working within a functional delivery model perform one specific set of tasks throughout the day. These tasks may include medication administration, assisting with activities of daily living, or developing the written plan of care. They are based upon the specific skill set of the individual performing the tasks, and within this particular model, workers can typically perform their assigned tasks without having to worry about influence or information from others performing their functions. In fact, this model was designed to improve efficiency by having nurses focus on just one set of tasks (Deutschendorf 2010).

In an open system there is continuous interaction with the outside environment. Essential components of an open system include inputs (resources), processes, outputs (products or services), and feedback (Greene 2005). Leaders in open systems are aware of what is going on all around. They continually assess what happens within and outside their system, seek feedback about their environment, and adjust processes as needed. Viewing an organization as an open system helps us to move away from "twentieth century work," where everything is done and viewed as separate, and move towards "twenty-first century work," where processes, ideas, and change overlap and integrate (Porter-O'Grady and Malloch 2011).

Organizations that use shared governance models are examples of open systems. The shared governance model flattens the traditional organizational hierarchy and focuses on empowering employees, gathering feedback at all levels, and solving problems where they occur in the organization (Smith 2010). The vision, goals, and operations are influenced by internal and external factors.

As industry and business began to grow rapidly in the early 1900s, many leaders and managers believed that organizations were in need of formalized structures and clear lines of authority in order to maximize efficiency and increase outputs (Meyer 2010). Under these rigid frameworks, process or quality improvements were often initiated from the top of the organizational chart and moved down with little to no input from the individuals at the bottom. In effect, there were efforts to keep the systems controlled and closed. With rapid changes in healthcare delivery and the push from most disciplines to improve interprofessional collaboration, many nursing leaders have been forced to take a different view of the organizations in which they operate. Tasks can no longer be performed in a bubble with no influence from the outside. Further, in healthcare especially, we cannot assume that what we do in one system does not have an impact on other systems. Moreover, "in an increasingly globalized and interconnected economy, however, it's increasingly hard to embrace the closed systems model even the abstract," (Kettl 2015).

Organizational theories provide a context in which to view organizational operations. They provide a framework for viewing, interacting with, and making changes within an organization. Organizational theories have evolved much as the view of organizations themselves have; from viewing organizations as closed systems that require formal structure and processes to a more contemporary view of organizations as open and adaptive systems. Table 4.1 shows an evolution of selected organizational theories over time.

At the next CHC provider meeting, Maya brings up this issue and discovers that the other providers have had similar issues when referring for services at the hospital. The infusion center will not take patients without having a primary care provider within the system and the pain clinic is considering a similar model. The providers and the CEO decide to request a meeting with executives of the hospital to discuss their concerns and hopefully to brainstorm options that will serve the needs of their rural community. Maya is asked to take the lead in setting up the meeting and begins to prepare.

TABLE 4.1. *Evolution of Selected Organizational Theories.*

Organizational Theory	Description	View of Organizations
Bureaucratic (Weber)	Organizations are structured and hierarchical with clear guidelines for decision making.	Closed
Scientific Management (Taylor)	Focus is on productivity and efficiency by simplifying job duties based on worker capabilities. Supervisory relationships are required.	Closed
Classic Management (Fayol)	Fourteen Principles of Management focusing on ideas such as division of work to increase efficiency, clear lines of authority, equitable pay, and order.	Closed
Contingency (Lawrence and Lorsch)	There is no one way to structure an organization. This is dependent (contingent) on a variety of factors such as environment, people, and technology.	Open
New Science (Wheatley)	Organizations are adaptive, creative, and resilient.	Open

In the case study, Maya worked in one organization (CHC) that frequently interacted with another separate organization (hospital system). While there was a cordial working relationship, it was clear the hospital viewed itself as a closed system when making decisions about referrals from outside organizations. The ripple effects of that decision outside the closed system of the hospital organization were not considered. Maya, on the other hand, considered both the CHC and the hospital as open systems that must (and already do) interact with one other. She also saw immediately that what happens in one system impacts another. She tried to call attention to the issue and make change but, unfortunately, met resistance. This did not dissuade her though. She persisted because she believed that she could influence change from within any level of an organization.

Systems Thinking

In 2001, The Institute of Medicine (IOM) called for an increase in systems thinking and a reengineering of how we envision healthcare. Systems thinking includes the ability to understand how one component in an organization or system impacts another. It allows us to recognize the steps necessary to make all of the parts of an organization or system work as one. It also helps us to understand how occurrences in one organization affect other organizations and perhaps the larger healthcare system of which they are a part. Unfortunately, more than 10 years later, many systems have made little to no efforts toward utilizing a systems thinking approach. Even more confounding is an apparent lack of preparation by healthcare leaders entering the field who are the leaders within the organization.

The field of systems thinking is not new and has been embraced for many years by other disciplines such as engineering and aerospace. Initially, systems thinking was conceived in the 1950s as a way to think about problems or innovation. It is a shift from a typical analysis in which a problem or issue is broken down to smaller and smaller parts. Rather, systems thinking was used to expand our view and encourage us to look outside the silos that are typical of bureaucratic organizations. Instead of a top-down approach, systems thinking allows us to consider the ripple effects that a decision has on one part of the system and how it may affect another. It also allows for a reflection of the potential unintended consequences (good or bad) of an action.

Systems theory borrows from biology in its comparison of organizations to living organisms. Each is made of systems that require inputs from the environment which are processed in some way, and a product is then produced. Systems theory also incorporates a sociological perspective that assumes humans are moral beings, and often seek to have a purpose beyond them within the organization. Thus, contemporary organizational leaders must consider the mindset of the twenty-first century employee. Pink (2005) affirms this, noting that employees are increasingly demanding a workplace to offer "meaning as well as money." Similarly, Jacobson (2000) addresses that building community in the workplace is integral to a successful organization. He explains that many organizations are learning that success requires a workforce that is "flexible, nimble, adaptable, and able to integrate diverse functions," (Jacobson 2000). In order to attract this type of employee, organizations need to provide a place where they find meaning and "collect more than a paycheck," (Jacobson 2000). As an organizational system is more open, input will be solicited and appreciated from all levels, and employees will be empowered to participate in decision making and change. This in turn will help the organization to attract and retain employees.

Finally, systems thinking also helps actors to take into account all the systems, at every level, that influence healthcare. These include micro-, macro-, and megasystems. A microsystem can be defined as a small group of individuals who routinely work together (The Dartmouth Institute 2013). In healthcare, the microsystem is the interface between the patient and his support systems and care givers (Cassel 2010). At the macro level, we find the organizations of which the microsystems are the building blocks. These include hospitals, clinics, or long-term care facilities. Finally, there is the concept of the megasystem. This is the larger healthcare delivery system within which the macro- and microsystems operate. The United States healthcare system is an example of a megasystem. All macrosystems must navigate and operate within this megasystem. Change in the megasystem, such as the Affordable Care Act (ACA), affect and have unintended consequences on both the macro- and microlevels. Anyone who has had to contend with implementing EHRs can attest to the ripple effects caused by changes within the megasystem. Similarly, changes at the microsystem or macrosystem levels can have an effect on the megasystem. For example, when patients use the emergency room for primary care services, this action in the microsystem puts strain on both the hospital system (macro) and the overall healthcare system (mega) by increasing costs.

Nursing leaders must be prepared to navigate an ever changing and complex healthcare delivery system. In order to do this, "advanced practice nursing leadership must acknowledge that the healthcare system is an open system, affected by, and to some degree dependent upon, larger systems of which it is a part," (Petersen 2011). Systems thinking in healthcare requires an investigation of how each level interacts

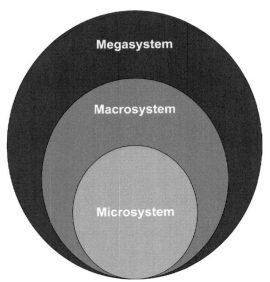

FIGURE 4.1.

with each other as well as how separate systems on each level (two separate nursing units within the same macrosystem). It is the interaction of these levels that provides either the continuity of patient care or fragmentation.

Despite her frustrations, Maya knows that she needs to try to understand why the hospital policy exists. She applies a systems thinking approach in order to understand the complexity of the issue. She brainstorms a few ideas on her own and gathers data from patients and her colleagues. She concludes that keeping patients within the same system for all their care has some obvious cost and safety benefits including efficient use of time, streamlining care, and ensuring adequate communication and follow up. Maya also knows there are a variety of consequences related to this policy that may not be beneficial to the hospital. She gathers data from her colleagues at the CHC, as well as patient stories who have been affected by this rule. Providers are feeling frustrated by having to choose between sending their patients away and not providing the best possible care. They have already begun using other hospital services less because of this matter. Every patient where this has become an issue is uninsured and cannot afford the transportation or extra money that switching to a different primary care provider would cost. Maya knows that there are other potential concerns for the hospital if they continue to enforce this policy with the CHC patients including missed appointments, unpaid balances, and the likely increase in use of emergency services. She is easily able to make a case for the potential revenue lost due to this policy. Finally, she gathers crucial evidence which supports the use of primary care providers in rural areas in order to increase access and reduce health disparities.

In the case study, Maya utilized a systems thinking approach to identify the healthcare actors and the impact that the hospital system's policies would have on her separate CHC system. She was able to articulate the unintended consequences that their policy decision had on her clinic system as well as on the hospital. If the hospital leaders used a systems thinking approach during their initial decision making, they would have identified a variety of issues related to this policy and perhaps worked to come to some different conclusions.

As leaders make decisions and influence change in their organizations, there are some key concepts that need to be considered when facilitating systems thinking. Kaplan *et al.* (2013) suggested four stages of systems thinking for healthcare organizations. These included:

1. *Identification:* Identify the multiple elements involved in caring for patients and promoting the health of individuals and populations.
2. *Description:* Describe how those elements operate independently and interdependently.
3. *Alteration:* Change the design of organizations, processes, or policies to enhance the results of the interplay and engage in a continuous improvement process that promotes learning at all levels.
4. *Implementation:* Operationalize the integration of the new dynamics to facilitate the ways people, processes, facilities, equipment, and organizations all work together to achieve better care at lower cost.

During the meeting, Maya encourages the executives to identify the various external agencies that are involved in caring for patients. She helps to articulate how these separate organizations impact the hospital as well as how hospital decisions impact them; the interdependence. Through this simple process, the executive team rethinks their position related to utilization of specialty services and their hospital and revise the policy to include patients from outlying areas and related agencies like the CHC. Maya is especially pleased when she is asked to be a part of a task force made up of stakeholders from the hospital and the interrelated external systems as they plan to expand services into other rural areas.

PATIENT CENTERED CARE

Much in the way that systems thinking approaches encourage us to view issues from multiple perspectives and to consider the myriad of influences on an organization, patient centered care is a way of viewing patients in a similar light. Rather than focusing on a particular "part" or ailment, patient centered care offers a richer assessment of unique individuals interacting within a complex environment. Patients (and families) should be involved in and considered when making decisions that may affect their health. Rickert (2012) suggests that "effective care is generally defined by or in consultation with patients rather than by physician dependent tools or standards."

The IOM has identified patient centered care as a core component of quality health care. This is likely because it has been shown to improve relationships between patient and provider, to decrease health care costs, and to utilize resources effectively (AHRQ 2011). Many organizations have embraced the idea of patient centered care; however healthcare team members need to be more proactive and demonstrate effective patient care based on clinical outcomes.

> Maya asks her nurse to initiate a referral to the Coumadin clinic at the closest hospital system which is 50 miles away. The patient reluctantly agrees to get a consult—although she already is concerned about the costs. Upon requesting the consult, the clinic nurse learns that in order to access the Coumadin clinic services, the patient must have a primary care provider who works within the hospital system. They will not accept a patient from "outside" the system. Maya is surprised by this new rule since she has frequently collaborated with specialists at the hospital in order to provide high quality health care to her patients. She makes some calls herself to see if she can explain this patient's case and perhaps get an exception. She is met with immediate resistance and is again told that her patient will need to transfer her primary care to the hospital clinic system in order to utilize the Coumadin clinic services. Maya discusses the options with her patient, who refuses to leave the CHC as her primary care home.

In the case study, Maya has a variety of options. She could simply tell her patient that she needed to leave the CHC and to seek primary and specialty care at the hospital system because that was "how we do things"—the status quo. She could also opt to manage her patient without the resources and collaboration she is seeking—which may delay care or lead to complications. Instead, Maya choses to put the patient at the center of the decision. She laid out the options in an honest and forthright way. When her patient weighed in, Maya took action to facilitate the necessary change.

ORGANIZATIONAL CHANGE

Organizational change can be very complicated since most individuals within any organization are initially resistant to change. There have been many organizational theories related to change such as: Lewin's unfreeze-change-refreeze, Kotter's eight steps, and Rogers' diffusion of innovation. Diffusion of innovation (DOI) will be discussed here in further detail because it fits so well with organizational change due to its focus on innovation rather than behavior.

Rogers' Diffusion of Innovation

Everett Rogers published the DOI theory in 1962. The focus of the DOI theory is on adopting an innovation rather than changing a behavior. An innovation is an "idea or practice that is perceived as new by an individual . . ." (Rogers 2003).

According to Rogers, there are five stages involved in the decision making process related to adopting an innovation. These include:

1. *Knowledge:* Develop the awareness of innovation and have an idea of how it works.
2. *Persuasion:* Form an opinion which can be positive or negative favorable.
3. *Decision:* Choose to adopt or reject the innovation and engage in activities that reflect the decision.
4. *Implementation:* Use the innovation.
5. *Confirmation:* Evaluate the results of the innovation used.

Rogers (2003) also describes five attributes that affect an individual's decision to adopt or accept the innovation. These include: (1) *relative advantage* (Is the innovation better than the current practice?), (2) *compatibility* (Is the innovation consistent with values, previous ideas, and/or perceived needs?), (3) *complexity* or *simplicity* (How difficult or simple is the innovation to use?), (4) *trialability* (Can the innovation be experienced on a limited basis?), and (5) *observability* (Will the results of an innovation be viewable to potential adopters?). When one is trying to implement a change, it is important to ensure that individuals have a sense of the relative advantage, compatibility, and simplicity of the innovation. In addition, assurance that there will be time for trial as well as to observe results of the change will help to persuade opinions and ultimately influence decisions about whether or not to adopt a change.

Rogers also developed five categories of adopters based on innovativeness. Innovativeness being the amount of time it takes for an individual to adopt to the new ideas as compared to others in the system. The innovators and early adopters are opinion leaders and risk takers. These people will be the first to adopt an innovation. The early majority will adopt an innovation just before the average group member. The late majority are typically late to adopt but do respond to peer pressure. The laggards are last to adopt and are typically suspicious of innovation and change.

Rogers recommends ensuring that the innovation is introduced to the innovators and early adopters in the organization in order to ensure that others will be eager to use the innovation.

> At the meeting Maya takes the lead and is able to succinctly state CHC's concerns, the consequences to all parties, and to make suggestions for resolution. Because of her preparation she is able to field questions and provide evidence based rebuttals to any concerns. Maya also has had past experience working with members of the hospital board on various community organizational committees. She knew in advance who might be willing to adopt change and who might be more resistant. She was careful to make sure her presentation won over the early adopters.

In the case study, Maya utilized elements of the diffusion of innovation theory. She knew members of the hospital board from previously working on committees with them. She was able to identify the laggards and early adopters and tailored her presentation to get buy-in from the early adopters. She knew that by convincing the early adopters first, they would help influence the other members of the team.

IMPACT OF THE AFFORDABLE CARE ACT

As the ACA was implemented, there was a continued increasing number of patients entering the healthcare system; many of whom had not ever accessed the system. The numbers of patients, their needs, and patient acuity were greater than ever before in the history of the United States healthcare system. The reimbursement models have changed to move from a focus on quantity (numbers of patients) to quality; thus patient outcomes were increasingly important. Nursing leaders and other healthcare providers were continued to be asked to do more with less. Progress cannot be achieved from separate institutional silos; rather, health teams need to be developed to provide the best patient care possible within a healthcare system.

Advance practice nurses will continue to be called upon to fill the ever growing gap of qualified healthcare providers in our country. They are also being called upon to step into leadership and consultant roles at all levels of the healthcare system in order to ensure that the voice of nursing is considered when key decisions are being made. In addition to achieving competency in their clinical area of practice, APNs will also be expected to (among other things) provide population focused care, function in and lead interprofessional teams, evaluate quality measures, and advocate for institutional and governmental policy changes in order to increase access to improve patient care. Thus, it is important for APNs to embrace the theories that undergird organizational structures, systems thinking, and innovative change processes.

SUMMARY POINTS

- Organizations can be viewed as closed systems or open systems. Closed systems do not interact with their external environment. Open systems are continuously assessing their surroundings, gathering data, and managing change.
- Healthcare is made up of microsystems (where patient and nurse or provider interact), macrosystems (clinics, hospitals, and healthcare organizations), and megasystems (the United States healthcare systems). Each system has an influence on and affects each other.
- System thinking involves an awareness of each system and how it interacts with the other. It is also considering an action's consequences (good or bad) within, between, and throughout all levels of a system.
- Systems thinkers in healthcare keep patients and families at the center of care decisions.
- Implementing change requires knowledge that there will always be resistance. It is also important to ensure that individuals have a sense of the relative advantage, compatibility, and simplicity of an innovation before it is adopted.
- Many provisions of the Affordable Care Act present a variety of opportunities for APNs to highlight their unique skill set and to advocate for improved patient care.

REFERENCES

American Association of Colleges of Nursing. 2006. *The Essentials of Doctoral Education for Advanced Nursing Practice.* American Association of Colleges of Nursing.

Agency for Healthcare Research and Quality. 2010. *National Healthcare Disparities Report Rockville, MD: Agency for Healthcare Research and Quality.* http://www.ahrq.gov/research/findings/nhqrdr/nhdr10/index.html

Cassel, C.K. 2010. Aging: Adding complexity: Requiring skills. In Rouse W.B. and D.A. Cortese, Eds., *Engineering the system of healthcare delivery* (47–70) Amsterdam: IOS Press.

Deutschendorf, A.L. 2010. Models of Care Delivery. In Huber, D.L., Ed, *Leadership and Nursing Care Management, 4th ed.*, (401–424). Maryland Heights: Saunders-Elsevier.

Greene, J. 2005. *Public administration in the new century: a concise introduction.* Belmont, CA: Thomson-Wadsworth.

Huber, D.L. 2010. Mission Statements, Policies and Procedures. In Huber, D.L., Ed, *Leadership and Nursing Care Management, 4th ed.*, (387–400). Maryland Heights: Saunders-Elsevier.

Institute of Medicine. 2001. *Crossing the quality chasm: a new health system for the 21st century.* Washington, DC: National Academies Press.

Jacobson, R. 2000. *Leading for a change: How to master the five challenges faced by every leader* (119–120). New York: Routledge.

Kaplan, G., G. Bo-Linn, P. Carayon, P. Pronovost, W. Rouse, P. Reid, and R. Saunders. 2013. *Bringing a systems approach to health.* Discussion Paper, Institute of Medicine and National Academy of Engineering, Washington, DC. http://www.iom.edu/systemsapproaches

Kettl, D.F. 2015. *Politics of the administrative process, 6th ed.* (87). Los Angeles: Sage Publications.

Meyer, R. 2010. Organizational Structure. In Huber, D.L., Ed, *Leadership and Nursing Care Management, 4th ed.* (401–424). Maryland Heights: Saunders-Elsevier.

Petersen, S. 2011. Systems Thinking, Healthcare Organizations and the Advanced Practice Nurse Leader. In Zaccagnini, M.E. and K.W., Eds., *The Doctor of Nursing Practice Essentials* (37–59). Sudbury, MA: Jones and Bartlett.

Pink, D. 2005. *A whole new mind: Why right brainers will rule the future* (224). New York: Penguin Group.

Porter-O'Grady, T. and K. Malloch. 2011. *Quantum Leadership: Advancing Innovation, Transforming Health Care, 3rd ed.* Sudbury, MA: Jones and Bartlett.

Rickert, J. 2012. Patient centered care: What it means and how to get there. *Health Affairs Blog.* http://healthaffairs.org/blog/2012/01/24/patient-centered-care-what-it-means-and-how-to-get-there/

Smith, C.D. 2010. Decentralization and shared governance. In Huber, D.L., Ed., *Leadership and Nursing Care Management, 4th ed.*, (425–440). Maryland Heights: Saunders-Elsevier.

Stevens, K., 2013. The Impact of Evidence-Based Practice in Nursing and the Next Big Ideas. *The Online Journal of Issues in Nursing 18*(2) DOI: 10.3912/OJIN.Vol18No-02Man04

The Dartmouth Institute. 2013. http://www.clinicalmicrosystem.org/about/background/

Wheatley, M.J. 2006. *Leadership and the new science: Discovering order in chaotic world, 3rd ed.* San Francisco: Berrett-Koehler Publishers.

Understanding Leadership and the Role of Nurse Practitioners in Critical Care Settings

MARY M. WYCKOFF, PHD., NNP-BC, ACNP, BC, FNP-BC, CCNS, CCRN, FAANP

Chapter 5 defines the role of the acute care nurse practitioner in clinical practice. It includes a case study that demonstrates leadership and change theories associated with the application of concepts for nurse practitioners working in changing health environments.

Case Presentation

Caroline Ashman PHD., ACNP, BC is an acute care nurse practitioner who has been assigned to change practice in an intercity, teaching facility that has a 40 bed surgical intensive care unit (SICU). The unit has a 20% patient turnover daily, is fast paced, and is intense critical care. The past history includes athat this unithas been managed with interns, residents, fellows, and physicians who change every month, and specifically at the beginning of the physician year, June and July. During these change periods, there is an increase in medical errors, a decrease in quality of patient care, and an increase in length of stay. Caroline was tasked with leading change to promote quality and safety as part of the future vision of nursing.

Caroline realized that this would be a difficult task since the change would encompass interdisciplinary leadership teams. This vision entailed advancing nursing leadership at the bedside, aligning nursing and physicians, and moving an archaic system into functioning system with high technology. Accomplishing this goal would need exceptional leadership skills and staged change encompassing strong team development.

55

Caroline became the lead nurse practitioner of a group in which a position did not exist and was to be designed and built from the effect of the change. The components of the physician infrastructure were challenged by cutbacks in physician residency hours and the gap in coverage for critical timeframes. This statistical challenge led to delays in care and increased length of stay. Caroline investigated leadership attributes since her previous experience entailed nursing management at a unit level. Caroline investigated effective leadership traits, which included knowledge, charisma, high performance, effective problem solving processes, and influencing others to be a part of a collective effort to manage, develop, and shape the direction of the future healthcare delivery system.

Caroline began with nurses at the bedside and sought their feedback on how the flow of the unit could be facilitated to enhance nursing care at the bedside and facilitate patient care dynamics. The meetings encouraged the thought process and the development of the practice of advancing nursing care abilities at the bedside. Nurses felt empowered to participate and embraced the unit as their own. They were encouraged to be leaders of change to enhance practice and to develop a new era of advancing practice at the bedside.

Nurses were challenged with thinking outside their normal routine and expectations at the bedside and questioned how they felt their care could be enhanced to envision a nurse of the future. Nurses were actively engaged and questioned about what they considered would improve care at the bedside.

Individual issues were evaluated based on the nursing thought process on the delay to care and increased length of stay. The first barrier addressed was procedural delay. The number one issue identified was the delay in extubation. Their ideas of educating and advancing nursing practice were embraced through the development of a protocol for post op extubation following evaluation from a resident, fellow, or NP. This practice was further enhanced as other delays to patient care were evaluated by nurses and changes were instituted to facilitate better patient care.

Often nurses could determine the patient's need for central vascular access (CVA) sooner than other healthcare staff. There was a delay in direct patient care such as CVA access because of physician cut backs and the lack of NPs. Nurses requested to be able to place peripherally inserted central catheters (PICCs) to facilitate early central access and decrease length of stay, delay in care, and vascular infiltrates. As a result, there were less secondary complications due to PICC insertions versus internal jugular or subclavian access.

Caroline embraced their ideas and swiftly provided educational advancement, the development of SICU protocols, and facilitated research and data collection to follow outcomes and monitor length of stay. These were key interventions for a facilitative leader. Enhancing and embracing bedside advancement of nurses created allies for further development and acceptance of advanced practice nurses into the SICU. The development of an intensivist model of an acute care nurse practitioner (ACNP) practice group to manage an intensive, fast paced SICU were new concepts for development and change for this traditional and archaic teaching institution.

This change process required political finesse to facilitate an understanding with some of the more senior nursing staff and the attending physician group. Futher, in order to incorporate an ACNP practice, physicians had to be comfortable with understanding that there would be no decrease in the educational benefits for the interns, residents, and fellows. Rather, these interdisciplinary groups would have enhanced learning abilities and they would not be burdened with the minutia of managing a very fast paced unit, thus they could focus on individualized patient care. The fellows were grouped with ACNPs to understand the dynamics and management of the SICU, also collaborating with bedside nursing.

Caroline's next goal was the development of the intensivist model of ACNP practice. The intensivist model included the use of interdisciplinary teams that would cover the unit 24 hours per day for every day of the year. Comprehending the individual patient needs, calculating a safe patient ratio for ACNP practice, and including educational components for not only bedside nurses, but also daily education of physician orientation, monthly physician change, and incorporating interdisciplinary daily rounds to assure all patient needs were facilitated required not only detailed leadership skills, but also ongoing management and the development of an interdisciplinary teams and integrative practice.

Approximately 6 months into the development of the intensivist model program, Caroline had facilitated the growth of the ACNP group to eight ACNPs with an autonomous practice, advancement of bedside nursing, and enhancement of intern, fellow, and resident education. Caroline further decreased length of stay by a minimum of one day due to early extubation. Patient satisfaction improved along with family satisfaction. Residency and fellowship programs received improving evaluations, while nursing satisfaction further improved. All of the success was secondary to Caroline's ability to communicate and facilitate an infrastructure that was enhanced by facilitative leadership skills and incorporating healthcare team development. Within the next year, Caroline's success grew to the development of a 16-member ACNP intensivist group model so that every patient in the SICU had an ACNP responsible for their care 24 hours per day, 365 days per year.

ESSENTIAL LEADERSHIP BEHAVIORS

According to Kouzes and Posner (1987), leadership behaviors have commonalities that lead to success. Leadership behaviors focus on analysis of the issues and challenge the process, which is the critical key to improvement. Building a team is one of the challenging concepts, as it generally takes a village to create change in a rigid, archaic environment. Sharing the vision through words, examples, ideas, science, and data collection are some of the strong leadership behaviors that enable a successful team concept. Facilitating and enabling the growth and development of others provides the tools, methods, education, and ideas to change the current environment. Being available, role modeling, and developing the path are the tools for building a strong foundation for a strong team. Always remember a boss tells others what to do, but a leader demonstrates what is feasible and able to be achieved (Marquis and Huston 2012).

> Caroline began with nurses at the bedside and sought their feedback on how the flow of the unit could be facilitated to enhance nursing care at the bedside and facilitate patient care dynamics. The meetings encouraged the thought process and the development of the practice of advancing nursing care abilities at the bedside. Nurses felt empowered to participate and embraced the unit as their own. They were encouraged to be leaders of change to enhance of practice and to develop a new era of advancing practice at the bedside.
>
> Caroline further facilitated the growth of nurses at the bedside by facilitating abstracts and through presentations national and international, including publication while developing future management leaders by demonstrating leadership behaviors.

Leadership and Nursing Satisfaction

Leadership must be visionary and ahead of the change that is about to occur. Leaders must develop, change, and grow as healthcare advances, concepts change, skills and technologies advance, and the basic requirements change (Glazer and Fitzpatrick 2013; Northouse 2012;

Tappen 1995). Of critical importance is understanding that the essence of leadership is the ability to influence others and understanding that management is very different than leadership, as management is about a process and leadership is about people (Parkin 2010; Fletcher 2003).

According to Maslow (1998), leadership is more about empowering and giving control versus trying to control. All members of the team need to understand the goal, contribute to the vision, and be invested in the future. Leaders are inspirational and need to emulate the role model they believe is the visionary of their theory and belief model. Loretta Ford was a visionary and saw the practice of advanced nurses at the bedside years prior to the development and success of this innovative practice. Florence Nightingale was a true visionary, a strong leader before her time.

According to Bass and Riggio (2006), "Transformational leaders are those who stimulate and inspire followers to both achieve extraordinary outcomes and, in the process, develop their own leadership capacity. Transformational leaders assist followers grow and develop into leaders by responding to individual followers' needs by empowering them and by aligning the objectives and goals of the individual followers, the leader, the group, and the larger organization. Evidence has accumulated to demonstrate that transformational leadership can move followers to exceed expected performance, as well as lead to high levels of follower satisfaction and commitment to the group and organization."

> Nurses were challenged with thinking outside their normal routine and expectations at the bedside and questioned how they felt their care could be enhanced to envision a nurse of the future. Nurses were actively engaged and questioned about what they considered would improve care at the bedside.

Transformational Leadership

According to American Association of Nurse Assessment Coordination (2013), transformational leadership facilitates confidence and inspiration to others while promoting staff respect and loyalty by providing encouragement support and praise. Transformational leadership is compared to a democratic leader encouraging open communication and staff support for decisions. The focus surrounds quality improvement, system management, and team building versus individual mistakes. This coincides with the drive towards The Magnet Recognition Program®, which promotes quality in a setting that supports professional practice and identifies excellence in the delivery of nursing services. The focus is on best practice and pride in quality care services. The only options for a successful program are leaders who facilitate change and transformation.

As a transformational leader, there is a multigenerational side, which the leader must facilitate as coexistents today that never existed in past history. There are nurses in their sixties working alongside nurses in their twenties who are leaders with a mixture of beliefs, changes, and challenges. Just reviewing the history of charting in that forty plus year generational gap is difficult to close the images and space time continuum. Computers and electronic medical records were nonexistent 40 years ago! Now the gap must be closed as it is critical that all individuals are functional and fulfilling the patient care needs while meeting all the new requirements. Keeping and sustaining multigenerational nurses is difficult to achieve, therefore focus on leadership and meeting the needs of the bedside nurse, advance practice nurse, and patients are critical in sustaining the level of knowledge needed to provide evidence-based care and best practice (Bach and Ellis 2011; Barr and Dowding 2008; WHO 2008).

> Caroline had to address many of these issues and provide political finesse while facilitating change and adapting not only to the physician group but also to nurses who were very set in their ways; this was a difficult adjustment and change. This change process required political finesse to facilitate with some of the more senior nursing staff and the attending physician group to realize that advancing nursing practice at the bedside while incorporating an acute care NP (APN) practice would not decrease the educational benefits for the interns, residents and fellows, but enhance their learning abilities so they would not be labored with the minutia of management of a very fast paced unit and could focus on individualized patient care. The fellows were grouped with APNs to understand the dynamics and management of the SICU also collaborating with bedside nursing.

Effective Team Building

The most important critical skills nurses, physicians, advance practice nurses, and all health care professionals is how to form effective team units and how to be an exceptional and strong team member while being able to maintain any role indicated. The value of strong team work, clear team communication, and exchange of accurate and clear situational awareness have been documented to increase safety and effectiveness especially in critical care environments. These patients are critically ill in a dynamic environment requiring astute care management of very complex patients, with strict time management and sensory overload.

The eight characteristics of effective teams with facilitative leadership include (Stahl *et al.* 2009):

1. Establish a safe and effective environment for open communication.
2. Provide briefings (huddles) that are thorough, interesting, and that address the current issues, team coordination, and planning.
3. Be approachable and inclusive of all healthcare providers and potential team members and be available to members of other teams.
4. Provide a climate that is appropriate to the operational environment and patient criticality.
5. Have an attitude of inclusiveness where members are encouraged to ask questions regarding team actions, plans, and decisions.
6. Have an attitude where members speak up and state their information in an appropriate, assertive, persistent, and timely manner.
7. Clearly state and verbally acknowledge clinical decisions.
8. Coordinate activities to establish proper balance between leadership and team participation.

The major skill sets necessary to build effective teams are communication skills and effective leadership. Efficient and clear communication is essential in the management of critically ill patients. Communication is the foundation of strong leadership skills and team function. According to The Joint Commission (2003), statistics have identified that 67% of the root cause of sentinel events are the result of errors in communication between team members (Reason 2004, 2000). Difficult team concepts and lack of communication or lapses among members of healthcare teams have emerged as key factors in the occurrence of errors. In healthcare, understanding team dynamics and practicing functional team skills is an important aspect of avoiding errors in the management of critically ill patients, especially in intensive care environments. Failure to communicate critical information in the operating room occurs in approximately 30% of team exchanges (WHO 2009). Such failures lead to inefficiency, emotional tension, delays, resource waste, patient inconvenience, and procedural error, all of which decrease quality and lead to increased morbidity and mortality.

Caroline's next goal was the development of the ACNP practice creating the intensivist model of interdisciplinary teams and building the practice to ultimately cover 24 hours per day and every day of the year. Comprehending the individual patient needs calculating a safe patient ratio for ACNP practice, and including educational components for not only bedside nurses, but daily education of physician orientation, monthly physician change, and incorporating an interdisciplinary daily rounds to assure all patient needs were facilitated required not only detailed leadership skills, but also ongoing management and the development of an interdisciplinary teams and integrative practice.

Teamwork

The intensivist model of ACNP incorporation into interdisciplinary teams stresses that teams are made up of many people, but that teamwork concepts are the skill of the individual. Transformational leadership facilitates the development of teams by grouping individuals with similar objectives, but differing levels of expertise and multidisciplinary skills sets; therefore, communication improvement strategies are best seen as the framework for supporting improved team function. High performing teams exhibit a sense of collective efficacy and recognize that they are dependent upon each other, interdependent within multiple teams, and believe that when working together with transformational leaders and strong self-confidence as a group they can solve complex problems. Effective teams are led by compelling transformational leaders and the teams are dynamic, optimize their resources, engage in self-correction, compensate for each other by providing back-up behaviors, and reallocate functions as necessary. Effective teams can respond efficiently in high stress and time restricted environments, and highly functional teams recognize potential problems or dangerous circumstances and adjust their strategies accordingly (WHO 2009; Zwarenstein *et al.* 2009; Zwarenstein and Bryant 2000).

Good teamwork establishes and maintains group and individual situational awareness and provides mutual support. Key benefits of good teamwork include added knowledge and expertise available to confront situations and synergy of ideas and skills so that the combined expertise of the group is greater than any individual. Effective transformational leaders facilitate the foresight of situational awareness and share information, experiences, perceptions, and ideas to keep everyone ahead of the evolving clinical situation (Stahl *et al.* 2009).

In all aspects of healthcare, exceptional leadership skills build strong team care, which has been shown to be more effective than nonteam care. According to Stahl *et al.* (2009), there were documented impressive reductions in mortality, morbidity, and length of stay in patients after major operations after institution of a formally trained emergency teams. Their prospective cohort study shows a reduction in relative risk of 57.8% ($p < 0.0001$) for major complication, reduction in relative risk of postoperative death by 36.6% ($p < 0.0178$), and reduction of postoperative length of stay by 4 days ($p < 0.0092$). Observational studies in the operating room have consistently demonstrated that training clinicians in nontechnical and teamwork skills provide important safety nets. This Level II data supports the conclusion that team training improves trauma and ICU team performance and recognition of life-threatening injuries with reduction in death, adverse outcomes, and lengths of stay.

The secondary sequel of strong leadership are individual and team situational awareness, judgment, safety, resource preservation, and competitive advantage. This important set of skills has been emphasized in the medical literature also to optimize and manage workload and task assignments, clinical task planning, and review and critique strategies. Skills such as prebriefs and "time-outs," and post-procedure debriefs are critical safety initiatives to plan procedures and decrease near misses. These skills are an indispensable element of communication in the operating room and Level II data supports the conclusion that these skills enhance the performance of the operating team and patient outcomes.

Effective Leadership skills are crucial parts of team dynamics that have been repeatedly emphasized in the literature and supported by The Joint Commission. Critical care leaders perform three key functions; they provide strategic direction, monitor the performance of the team, and educate team members by providing education, all of which are models that match those that researchers identified in the functional team leadership literature. The characteristics of leadership in trauma teams has been studied by Yun *et al.* (2005) in a Level I trauma center. They stressed the importance of leadership adaptability since team leaders and their teams work in an uncertain and time-constrained environment. Trauma leaders cannot anticipate when critical patients will arrive or how many and what type of injuries they will face. They often do not know with accuracy such essential information as a patient's medical history and leadership adaptability becomes more important in uncertain and urgent situations. The ability to get the best performance from all team members and to encourage each person on the team to share information and knowledge are strong traits of exceptional leaders and supervisors that have been stressed in the literature (Stahl *et al.* 2009).

Approximately 6 months into the development of the intensivist model program Caroline had facilitated the growth of the APN group to eight APNs with an autonomous practice, advancement of bedside nursing, and enhancement of intern, fellow, and resident education. Caroline further decreased length of stay by a minimum of one day due to early extubation. Patient satisfaction improved along with family satisfaction. Residency and fellowship programs received improving evaluations, while nursing satisfaction further improved. All of the success was secondary to Caroline's ability to communicate and facilitate an infrastructure that was enhanced by facilitative leadership skills and incorporating health care team development.

Strong and effective transformational leadership skills build effective, well communicating team concepts which create safety tools adapted for use by critical care teams. These concepts facilitate a strong role in capturing and preventing errors. Research based evidence shows that care delivered through team concepts is more effective and decreases errors, mortality, and morbidity while preventing adverse events in healthcare (Stahl *et al.* 2009; WHO 2009; The Joint Commission 2008).

SUMMARY POINTS

- An understanding of the importance of leadership behaviors are necessary to promote change in clinical settings.
- Nursing and nursing satisfaction are linked to provide safe, effective patient care practice.
- Transformational leadership provides an understanding of effective teamwork.
- Teamwork must be valued and each team member needs to be aware of how they influence the ability of the team to function.
- Use of the intensivist model of acute care nurse practitioner (ACNP) practice group enhanced patient outcomes in one medical center's SICU.
- Use of a transformational leadership model provides an effective platform for safe and effective clinical care.

REFERENCES

Bach, S. and P. Ellis. 2011. *Leadership, Management and Team working in Nursing. Learning Matters.* Exeter.

Barr, J. and L. Dowding. 2008. *Leadership in Health Care.* London: Sage.

Bass, B. 1985. *Leadership and Performance Beyond Expectations.* New York: Free Press.

Bass, B. and R. Riggio. 2006. *Transformational Leadership, 2nd ed.* Lawrence Erlbaum Associates, Mahwah, New Jersey.

Fletcher, J.K. 2003. The Paradox of Post Heroic Leadership: Gender Matters (Working Paper, No. 17). Boston: Center for Gender in Organizations, Simmons Graduate School of Management.

Glazer, G. and J. Fitzpatrick. 2013. *Nursing leadership from the outside in NY,* Springer Publishing.

Kouzes, J. and B. Posner. 1987. The Leadership Challenge. San Francisco: Jossey-Bass. The Magnet Recognition Program® http://www.nursecredentialing.org/magnet.aspx

Marquis, B. and C. Huston. 2012. *Leadership Roles & Management Function in Nursing. Theory & Application, 4th ed.* Philadelphia: Lippincott, Williams & Wilkins.

Maslow, A. 1998. *Maslow on Management.* John Wiley & Sons, Inc., New York

Northouse, P.G. 2012. *Introduction to Leadership: Concepts and Practice, 2nd ed.* Thousand Oaks CA: Sage Publications.

Parkin, S. 2010. *The Positive Deviant. Sustainability Leadership in a Perverse World.* Chapter 4. Earthscan. London.

Reason, J. 2000. Human Error: models and management (768–70). *BMJ* 320.

Reason, J. 2004. Beyond the organizational accident: the need for "error wisdom" on the frontline. *Quality and Safety in Health Care; 13*:ii (28–33).

Stahl, K., A. Palileo, C. Schulman, K. Wilson, J. Augenstein, C. Kiffin, *et al.* 2009. Enhancing patient safety in the Trauma/Surgical intensive care unit. *Journal of Trauma, 67*, 430–5.

Tappan, R.M. 1995. *Instructor's Guide for Nursing Leadership and Management Concepts, 3rd ed.* Davis Company.

The Joint Commission. 2003. http://www.jointcommission.org/core_measure_sets.aspx

World Health Organization. 2008. Closing the gap in a generation. Health equity through action on the social determinants of health.

World Health Organization. 2009. *Guidelines for Safe Surgery 2009: Safe Surgery Saves Lives.* http://www.ncbi.nlm.nih.gov/books/NBK143239/

Yun, S., S. Faraj, and H.P. Sims. 2005. Contingent leadership and effectiveness of trauma resuscitation teams (90, 1288–96). *Journal of Applied Psychology.*

Zwarenstein M. and W. Bryant. 2000. Interventions to improve collaboration between nurses and doctors. In: Bero, L., R. Grilli, J. Grimshaw, A. Oxman, and M. Zwarenstein, Eds. *Cochrane Collaboration on effective professional practice module of the Cochrane database of systematic reviews. In: Cochrane Collaboration. Cochrane Library. Issue 2.* Oxford: Update Software.

Zwarenstein, M., J. Goldman, and S. Reeves. 2009. Interprofessional collaboration: effects of practice based interventions on professional practice and healthcare outcomes. *Cochrane Effective Practice Review Group.* DOI: 10.1002/14651858.CD000072.pub2

Leadership in the Clinical Setting

JACQUELINE ROBERTS DNP, FNP-BC, AOCNP

The Chapter 6 case study emphasizes the role of the advanced practice nurse in the clinical setting. Topics include the transition to a leader in the clinical setting, the characteristics of a clinical leader, quality and safety issues as an APN leader, and potential challenges of a clinical leader.

Case Presentation

Dr. Dieson DNP, FNP is a nurse practitioner at Primary Care Associates (PCA) in rural Montana. Recently, he relocated with his family to a rural setting and has worked in primary care for the past 10 years. PCA employs a part time family practice physician, two full time nurse practitioners, a certified nurse midwife, a part time physical therapist, a pharmacist, and a dietician. The primary care physician has worked at PCA for 27 years and has assumed many administrative duties. The nurse practitioner is a new grad and has lived within the community her entire life and is well connected with community members.

Dr. Dieson's previous experience allowed him to feel comfortable managing acute and chronic health conditions as well as health promotion and education. Throughout his education and work experience he has had the ability to provide leadership on a small scale in small groups within his unit. The first few months of his new position at PCA he spent the majority of his time getting to know the clinic staff and providers as well as other professionals in the community. He felt he was developing a good rapport with the community members and was starting to feel vested in the community. Thus far, he has been able to assume dual relationships within the community and has gained acceptance from the community members.

Dr. Dieson was building his practice when he noticed that his patients who had a diagnosis of asthma were not following the national guidelines and recommendations for evidenced-based care. When he inquired with staff, they stated, "It has always been that way." Dr. Dieson did not want to offend his colleagues or staff, and knew that he had to handle this situation carefully. He began to think of bringing forward his concerns as an opportunity for change. Dr. Dieson remembered several processes through his DNP education that would be helpful during this time of transition. He recalled the necessary steps of completing a needs assessment, identifying key stakeholders, and the importance of "buy in" to the project. Dr. Dieson began to use evidence-based practice (EBP) guidelines with his patient encounters in practice. Colleagues and other providers took note of this in the clinical setting and in the EHR.

Dr. Dieson made sure he was aware of new policies at the state and federal levels that might impact his patients. He shared this information with coworkers and they began to take an interest and to view Dr. Dieson as a role model. Dr. Dieson was always willing to teach coworkers, he enjoyed opportunities to answer questions and to teach a new concept. He was easily approachable and had the ability to make colleagues and staff feel valued when they approached him with questions. Dr. Dieson was a hard worker in the clinical setting and coworkers took note of that and respected his work ethic.

Dr. Dieson concluded that it was important to initiate an EBP protocol for asthma care within the clinic. He involved the pharmacist who was well known in the community and took the time to complete these steps as well as preparing a budget and educational tools for providers, staff, and patients regarding evidenced-based asthma care. He outlined the benefits, cost savings, potential days missed from work or school, and the impact on quality of life. Throughout the planning and organization he gained tremendous support from colleagues, staff, and eventually patient and community members. He was able to implement the guidelines successfully.

Over the next several years he was able to identify areas of improvement in the clinical setting. Often, these areas were identified by a trigger or event that would allow him to reflect on the process, safety, quality, and outcomes of interventions (or lack thereof) that occurred in the clinical setting. One day in the practice setting, he observed a near fatal reaction to a medication that was not properly noted on the EHR. He immediately initiated and implemented a new process for reviewing patient's meds and allergies.

Over the next few days he noticed the staff was upset and he inquired with a nurse regarding staff morale. She reported that the staff felt as though it was their "fault" and they were disappointed in how quickly a process was initiated without their input. The staff did not feel there was a need for change; after all, the system had worked well for many years. Dr. Dieson quickly called a meeting to communicate the reasoning for a change in the process. He had a clear vision to improve safety and allowed employees to have input and to take on ownership of the process. He acknowledged how hard the staff worked and the positive attributes of the team. He also took responsibility for moving quickly without input for feedback from others within the clinic, but stressed the importance of safety and responsibility to patients. Dr. Dieson quickly learned to be aware of implications of change and anticipate potential barriers in the future.

Dr. Dieson was able to effectively work interprofessionaly with the physical therapist, pharmacist, and dietician in a collaborative team effort. He was keenly aware of what each discipline brought forward for patient outcome. By understanding and participating in interprofessional practice, health policy, and evidenced-based outcomes, he was able to meet the needs of his patients and the community. This had a positive impact on the quality of life in this rural community.

ROLE OF THE ADVANCED PRACTICE NURSE LEADER IN THE CLINICAL SETTING

Clinical leadership is defined as the direct involvement in clinical care while influencing others to improve the care they provide (Cook 1999). There is an obvious need for leaders in the clinical setting. The healthcare setting continues to change because of the rapid changes related to healthcare reform, the demand from consumers for quality care, and the demand for improved outcomes. Nurses will need leadership skills and competencies to act as full partners with physicians and other healthcare professionals (IOM 2010). In order to accomplish this task, leadership capacity and lifelong leadership development must be maximized in nursing education.

The APN is someone who has a direct care role and is certified as one of the following: Certified Registered Nurse Anesthetists (CRNA), Certified Nurse Midwife (CNM), Certified Nurse Specialist (CNS), or

Certified Nurse Practitioner (CNP). The APN traditionally works in a clinical setting with patients at the point of care; typically one-on-one care that occurs during a patient encounter. In an ideal setting, the APN is part of an interdisciplinary team who has direct influence on patient care, safe quality care, as well as patient outcomes. The unique perspective of an APN allows him to see the effects of the organizational development and processes at the point of care. The ability to deliver one-onone care to patients, families, and the community allows the APN to reflect on the healthcare system and the possible need for change. In 2011, Cook concluded that a clinical leader was most likely to be "a nurse involved in providing clinical care." This unique opportunity gives the APN a perspective that will allow them to suggest change in order to improve patient outcomes overall.

The profession of nursing suffers from differing opinions on the definition of leadership versus management. Leadership has been defined as the process of helping individuals, departments, or organizations adapt to change (Jacobson 2000). Leadership has the ability to help people think outside the box and to move an organization forward. The leader is keenly aware of the needs of the organization and community as well as the financial resources available to the organization. The leader promotes professional and collaborative teamwork as well as demonstrates role model behavior for employees. A manager, however, delegates responsibility, plans for performance of the organization, allocates resources, and is responsible for results and outcomes (Jacobson 2000). Managers typically receive "on the job training;" they understand hiring and complete performance reviews and budgets as a large part of their role. Managers typically have worked with and managed small groups of people.

Leadership in the clinical setting may take on many forms and is not necessarily someone who has a leadership title; rather, it may be someone who is well respected or viewed by others as a role model. In the case study, Dr. Dieson takes on a leadership role without a formal title. He is in a role where he provides point of care with the patient. This allows Dr. Dieson to have a greater understanding of patient outcomes and the need for change. Because of his clinical experience and education, he is prepared to evaluate the needs of the community and clinic so that he may assume a leadership role.

Historically, nurse leaders have been promoted because they have excelled in their position as a clinician. New APN graduates often aspire to be clinicians; few transition to practice with the intent of becoming nurse leaders (Scott and Miles 2013). In this type of role they have adopted leadership styles by observation and informally learning from other leaders. Nurse leaders in the clinical setting tend to evolve a leadership style based on experience and the management of patient groups.

LEADERSHIP IN HEALTH SYSTEMS

In order to understand the impact a leader can have on a health system, the different levels of the system must first be understood. The APN may participate in leadership on a micro-, macro-, or megalevel. The nurse leader is aware of the systems and organization as they lead their employees through change. The interface between the patients and their caregivers is considered a microlevel of the health system. It is the patient/provider interaction; or it may be a place, a provider's office, emergency room, or urgent care facility and the day-to-day activities that occur within that space. In the case study, an example of the microsystem is the provider's office where one-on-one care takes place with the patient, provider, nurse, and family. The macrolevel is the organization itself, the hospital, institutions, or clinics that compose the microsystem. An example if a macrosystem within this case study is PCA since it is the organization that houses the microsystem. If we take this one step further we can consider the megalevel as the healthcare delivery system as a whole: healthcare within the state of Montana and the outcomes associated with rural primary care. The micro- and macrolevels are within the megasystem. Another consideration at the megalevel is the relationship to the affordable care act; this is healthcare at a larger level, nationally or globally. It is important that the nurse leader is aware of the systems level and the interaction between all three levels. The leader must be mindful of all levels and resources at each level.

TRANSITION TO ADVANCED PRACTICE NURSE LEADERSHIP IN CLINICAL SETTINGS

Transition and change can be a difficult task in any situation. An APN may find the transition to leadership in the clinical setting overwhelming. An APN may be comfortable in the role of clinician or provider, but when faced with leadership responsibilities, the new role may seem daunting.

Dr. Dieson was busy building his practice when he noticed that his patients who had a diagnosis of asthma were not following the national guidelines and recommendations for evidences-based care. When he inquired with staff, they stated, "It's always been that way." Dr. Dieson did not want to offend his colleagues or staff,

TABLE 6.1. Kouzes and Posner Leadership Practice and Commitment.

Leadership in Principles	Characteristics
Modeling the way	Establish principles concerning the way people should be treated and the way goals should be pursued.
Inspiring a shared vision	Envision the future and create and invite others to share in the vision.
Challenging the process	Search for opportunities by looking for innovative ways to improve.
Enabling others to act	Foster collaboration by building relationships and strengthen others by encouraging self-determination and competence.
Empowering the heart	Appreciate others and celebrate values by creating a spirit of community.

and knew that he had to handle this situation carefully. He began to think of bringing forward his concerns as an opportunity for change.

Successful transition requires knowledge, skills, tools, and resources to achieve the desired goal. A good leader is aware of his own leadership style as well as his strengths and weaknesses as a leader. This self-awareness allows leaders to recognize their own emotions, needs, and drives (Goleman 1998). It allows them to have an understanding of their values and goals. Often, leaders are motivated beyond monetary reimbursement. A leader is driven by the desire to produce change. Kouzes and Posner (2011) describe a structure five-stage model of exemplary leadership practices (Table 6.1). These key concepts are defined as desirable characteristics or practices in which a leader can motivate staff.

In the case study, Dr. Dieson demonstrates many desirable concepts of a leader by acting as a role model to employees and by sharing a vision of a healthier community with positive health outcomes. Dr. Dieson challenges the process by asking the question regarding EBP and by initiating EBP protocols. Dr. Dieson was able to empower staff by involving them in the process, seeking input, and allowing them to be a part of the process.

CHARACTERISTICS OF A CLINICAL LEADER

One can assume there are many characteristics that may be desirable in the clinical leader. Advanced nurse leaders are role models for their staff and colleagues. They demonstrate professional behavior that others look up to and aspire to become. Advanced nurse leaders must be educated and knowledgeable within their specialty and at the same time must be keenly aware of limitations. They work interprofessionally to achieve the best outcomes. They are aware of policy at the local, state, and federal level and how policy can impact their patients and community. Advanced nurse leaders are good communicators; they are able to use clear and concise communication in order to effectively work with others. They are approachable, fair, and trustworthy. This allows them to be respected in their specialty area within their work environment.

> Dr. Dieson made sure he was aware of new policies at the state and federal levels that might impact his patients. He shared this information with coworkers and they began to take an interest and to view Dr. Dieson as a role model. Dr. Dieson was always willing to teach coworkers; he enjoyed opportunities to answer questions and to teach a new concept. He was easily approachable and had the ability to make colleagues and staff feel valued when they approached him with questions. Dr. Dieson was a hard worker in the clinical setting and coworkers took note of that and respected his work ethic.

Leaders who are active and working in the clinical setting are often seen as hard working and vested in the organization and the daily work of the clinical setting. They take into consideration what needs to be done on a daily basis for the organization to function. They are motivated and have a goal in sight, which others may find motivating. Nurse leaders provide a safe environment for staff, colleagues, and patients to approach them with questions or concerns.

In the case study, Dr. Dieson demonstrates many of these characteristics since he is fair and trustworthy. He utilized role modeling and demonstrated professional behaviors consistent with his widespread clinical knowledge. Employees are able to approach him with questions and he is always willing to teach new concepts. Dr. Dieson is able to empower others, which helps to ensure "buy in," which in turn, allows for the employees to feel valued and committed to the vision of the organization or department.

LEADERSHIP STYLES

There are many different types of leaders defined in literature. This chapter focuses on leadership styles which are described as transactional, transformational, or situational leadership. Transactional leaders are described as individuals who offer rewards to employees for compliance and provide positive reinforcement based on the employee's performance. The transactional leaders develop management tasks and often are not seen as team players since they are viewed as autocratic, controlling, and power orientated. On the other hand, transitional leaders focus on motivating others and may encourage staff to envision and achieve change (Bass and Avolio 1993). This type of leader communicates effectively to all staff and provides consistent and clear communication.

Transformational leaders inspire their employees to go above and beyond since they act as mentors. They improve their employee's self-esteem, and stress motivation and job satisfaction. They have a clear vision of the future and demonstrate qualities of a democratic type of leader (Giltinane 2013).

Last, a situational leader is defined as a leader who is supportive and has directive behaviors based on the event or occurrence (Grimm 2010). There may be times when the situation defines the type of leadership necessary to move forward, thus depending on the event, the leader adapts the leadership style to fit the situation.

> Dr. Dieson began to use EBP guidelines with his patient encounters in practice. Colleagues and other providers took note of this in the clinical and in the EHR. Dr. Dieson made sure he was aware of new policies at the state and federal levels that might impact his patients. He shared this information with coworkers and they began to take an interest and to view Dr. Dieson as a role model. Dr. Dieson was always willing to teach coworkers, he enjoyed opportunities to answer questions and to teach a new concept. He was easily approachable. Dr. Dieson was a hard worker in the clinical setting and coworkers took note of that and respected his work ethic.

Dr. Dieson displayed characteristics consistent with a transformational leadership style. His ability to be a good role model, mentor, and teacher facilitated the employee's ability to improve their self-esteem. Dr. Dieson expressed a clear vision of improving the health of the community and sought input from employees thus allowing them to be an active part of the process.

However, when Dr. Dieson was faced with a near fatal error, he displayed characteristics of a transactional leader with autocratic qualities. He received resistance from employees and had difficulty moving forward with a new process. Sometime leaders will need to assess the situation and adapt the leadership style that best reflects the situation. In this instance, Dr. Dieson felt compelled to act quickly for safety issues. Perhaps a blended form of transaction and transformational leadership would have been more effective.

LEADERSHIP TO INFLUENCE QUALITY AND SAFETY

APNs are aware of quality and safety issues within an organization and they ensure safety standards are considered when proposing a change. Clinical leadership involves the difficult process of managing patients, taking into consideration economic constraint while promoting quality improvement and patient safety (Scott and Miles 2013). Clinical leadership has been describes as having five dimensions: clinical expertise, effective communication, collaboration, coordination, and interpersonal understanding (Patrick *et al.* 2011).

> Over the next several years he was able to identify areas of improvement in the clinical setting. Often, these areas were identified by a trigger or event that would allow him to reflect on the process, safety, quality, and outcomes of interventions (or lack thereof) that occurred in the clinical setting. One day in the practice setting he observed a near fatal reaction to a medication that was not properly noted on the EHR.

In the case study, Dr. Dieson displayed clinical expertise; he was able to utilize his 23 years of experience and make changes based on expertise. Dr. Dieson displayed good communication and clear and concise goals when initialing EBP for asthma care. Dr. Dieson was able to work collaboratively with the pharmacist and coordinate an effective EBP for asthma care within the clinic.

CHALLENGES OF A LEADER IN THE CLINICAL SETTING

The need for advanced nursing leadership in the clinical setting is evident now more than ever. The clinical setting provides many opportunities for change, but change can be a difficult process. Portoghese *et al.* (2012) found that nurses are more likely to commit to change if they have positive expectations regarding the recommended changes. One major challenge is fear of change by employees. As demonstrated in the case study, the nursing staff did not want to change. It is important for leaders to build relationships, communicate effectively, and to share the same vision and goals as staff and coworkers.

Challenges include preparation of clinical leadership as well as a clear definition about the characteristics of a clinical leader. The need for leadership education is necessary if we want to promote an advanced practice clinical leader. Teaching strategies for leadership differ in the academic setting and there is no consensus on evidenced-based strategies for teaching leadership (Curtis *et al.* 2011).

TABLE 6.2. *Jacobson's Five Key Leadership Challenges (2000).*

Leadership Steps	Definition
Reframe the future	Develop a new set of possibilities.
Develop commitment	Develop employees who are willing to address changes eagerly, honestly, and openly.
Teach and learn	Encouraging learning.
Build a community	Consider culture, infrastructure, and governance.
Balance paradox	Learn to cope with paradox and develop balanced view of situation.

There are many potential challenges leaders may face. Table 6.2 (Jacobson 2000) describes five key leadership challenges ranging from reframing the future to balancing leadership situations.

A leader must be able to understand the organizational dynamics and be able to reframe the future within the organizational context. This reframing allows the leader and key players to consider a new vision or change for the organization. A second challenge is commitment from leaders, colleagues, and staff. Staff and coworkers may begin to feel vested in the organization if the leader is able to empower them, make them part of a team, and create diversity within the team. If a leader is able to promote an environment of teaching and learning where staff may feel committed to the mission of the organization, the change can begin to occur. Some ways that this can be accomplished may include sending staff to conferences on leadership or specialty conferences in relation to their expertise or appointing them as leaders of a team or part of an interdisciplary team. This feeds into the development of a community from all key stakeholders and develops the values and common goals for all those involved. Finally, all organizations have difficulties from time to time and this period of conflict can be viewed as a paradox. A paradox occurs when two views are distinctly opposite at the same time (Jacobson 2011). These views do not need to be managed as conflict; rather a balance between the two should be considered to explore a variety of resolutions that are acceptable to all parties.

One barrier to overcome includes resistance to change since some employees don't like change and are unwilling to accept the changes. A second barrier may be lack of resources. Thus, in order for change to occur, resources must be part of the solution. Last, the leader may have the ability to influence others or employees may not view the person proposing change as a leader. Often, these barriers impact the culture of the organization's ability to effectively change.

Over the next few days he noticed the staff was upset and he inquired with a nurse regarding staff morale. The nurse reported that the staff felt as though it was their "fault" and they were disappointed in how quickly a process was initiated without their input. The staff did not feel there was a need for change; after all, the current system had worked well for many years. Dr. Dieson quickly called a meeting to communicate the reasoning for a change in the process. He had a clear vision to improve safety and allowed employees to have input and take on ownership of the process. He was sure to acknowledge how hard the staff worked and the positive attributes of the team. He also took responsibility for moving quickly without input for feedback from others within the clinic. Dr. Dieson quickly learned to be aware of implications of change and to anticipate potential barriers.

In this case, Dr. Dieson initiated an immediate new process for reviewing medications and allergies. Employees did not have a clear understanding of the need for change. When Dr. Dieson was able to explain the process, have a clear vision, and include the employees in the process, he was able to move forward. Thus, change was initiated once all members in the organization were involved in understanding the outcomes associated with the change.

CLINICAL PRACTICE LEADERS OF THE FUTURE

Advanced Nurse Leaders have great opportunity to be instrumental in developing a practice environment to bridge the gap from fragmented care to multidisciplinary care (IOM 2010). The APN clinician has the ability to evoke system changes and processes and to improve patient outcomes at the point of care. Nurses should be prepared to assume leadership positions across all levels of care (IOM 2010). Nurse leaders of the future will use their education and experience to influence healthcare organizations. They will look to the future for new and innovative ways to provide healthcare, enhance relationships, and establish buy-in from key stakeholders.

Nurse-led clinics are one example of a practice model that has occurred as a result of the accepted role of the APN. Nurse-led clinics demonstrate good outcomes and contribute to containing healthcare costs (Wong and Chung 2006). The role of the APN as a clinical leader may expand into leadership positions within the organization, such as CEO or president of hospitals, clinics, or health centers. The Doctorate of Nursing Practice prepares APNs for these future roles.

Dr. Dieson was able to effectively work interprofessionaly with the physical therapist, pharmacist, and dietician in a collaborative team effort. He was keenly aware of each discipline brought forward for each patient outcome. By understanding and participating in interprofessional practice, health policy, and evidenced-based outcomes, he was able to meet the needs of his patients and the community. This had a positive impact on the quality of life in this rural community.

SUMMARY POINTS

- The healthcare environment is rapidly changing, and the demand for leaders in the clinical setting is evident now more than ever.
- Characteristics of leaders in the clinical setting include being a good role model, well respected, professional, fair, and trustworthy.
- Leadership in the clinical settings is essential to providing evidenced-based care, improving healthcare systems, and providing better patient and population health outcomes.
- There are many challenges that lie ahead for clinical leaders, and it will be important for leaders to overcome these barriers and challenges.
- Clinical practice leaders of the future will work interprofessioanly to improve the delivery of healthcare. Additionally, the future clinical practice leader will be essential in the overall improvement of patient and population health outcomes.

REFERENCES

Bass, B. and B. Avolio. 1993. Transformational leadership and organizational culture. *Public Administration Quarterly. 44*(3), 112–121.

Cook, M.J. 1999. Improving care required leadership in nursing. *Nurse Education Today, 19*(4), 306–312.

Cook, M.J. 2001. The renaissance of clinical leadership. *International Nursing Review, 48*(1), 38–46. doi:10.1046/j.1466-7657.2001.00040.x

Curtis, E.A., F.K. Sheerin, and J. deVines. 2011. Developing Leadership in Nursing; Exploring Core Factors. *British Journal of Nursing. 20*(5), 306–309.

Goleman, D. 1998. What Makes a Leader? *Harvard Business Review, 93.* Retrieved from http://go.galegroup.com.ezproxy.undmedlibrary.org/ps/i.do?id=GALE%7CA53221401&v=2.1&u=ndacad_58202zund&it=r&p=EAIM&sw=w&asid=61a58bd6702911b67e92c78b1ca83ab8

Giltinane, C.L. 2013. Leadership Styles and Theories. *Nursing Standard. 27*(41), 35–39.

Grimm, J.W. 2010. Effective leadership: making the difference. *Journal of Emergency Nursing. 36*(1), 74–77.

Institute of Medicine (IOM). 2010. *The Future of Nursing: Leading change, advancing health.* Washington, DC: The National Academies Press.

Jacobson, R. 2000. *Leading for a Change.* Boston, MA: Butterworth Heinmann.

Kelly, L., T. Wicker, and R. Gerkin. 2014. *Journal of Nursing Adminstration 44*(3), 158–163.

Kouzes, J. and B. Posner. 2011. *The Five Principles of Exemplary Eldership, 2nd ed.* San Francisco, CA: Pfieiffer.

Patrick, A., H. Laschinger, C. Wong, and J. Finegan. 2011. Developing and testing a new measurement of staff nurse clinical leadership: the clinical leadership survey. *Journal of Nurse Management. 19*: 449–460.

Portoghese, I., M. Galletta, A. Battistelli, L. Saiaiani, M.P. Penna, and E. Allegrini. 2012, Change-related expectations and commitment to change of nurses: the role of leadership and communication. *Journal of Nursing Management, 20*: 582–591. doi: 10.1111/j.1365-2834.2011.01322.x

Scott, E. and J. Miles. 2013. Advancing leadership capacity in nursing. *Nursing Administration Quarterly. 37*(1), 77–82.

Wong F. and L. Chung. 2006. Establishing a definition for nurse led clinic; structure, process and outcome. *Journal of Advanced Nursing. 53.* 358–369.

Defining Quality Patient Care

JUDITH SELTZER MS, BSN, RN, CNOR

Chapter 7 presents two short, critical thinking case studies to assist the APN with an understanding of how to implement change in a healthcare setting that promotes quality patient outcomes.

Although there is a plethora of knowledge combined with experience to review, analyze, enhance strategies, and promote change, questions still arise over the global quality of healthcare. Change requires healthcare professionals to think differently and provide new ways to approach patient care. Although the healthcare facility or system is well developed and based on a wide variety of standards of care, the expected outcomes of quality patient care is not achieved. A newsletter addressing the Institute of Medicine's forum, *Crossing the Quality Chasm: A New Health System for the 21st Century*, reflects the following:

As medical science and technology has advanced at a rapid pace, the healthcare delivery system has floundered in its ability to provide consistently high quality care to all. Healthcare systems do not use all of their resources effectively (IOM 2001).

Presently, there are more than 70 global health partnerships (WHO 2006). Although many of these initiatives have brought considerable improvement to many countries, there is still an opportunity to improve the quality of care and performance of those persons, facilities, or systems that provide healthcare.

Often, healthcare personnel are reluctant to embrace change since they are used to providing care based on a fee for service model versus the quality indicators associated with patient outcomes. However, as healthcare reimbursement models demand patient centered outcomes, healthcare providers will have to make the necessary changes to compete.

81

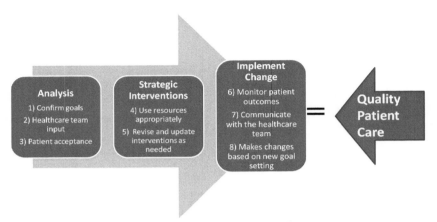

FIGURE 7.1. Strategy to implement change.

APNs, whether they are nurse practitioners, clinical nurse specialists, nurse anesthetists, or nurse midwives, play a pivotal role in the future of healthcare. APNs are often primary care providers and are at the forefront of providing preventative care to the public. To be effective, they must be grounded in didactic theory as well as have a strong preparation to clinical practice. Although their primary focus is their patient, APNs must also effectively communicate and collaborate with multiple members of the patient's overall healthcare team. APNs are tasked to optimize their resources in order to integrate strategic measures that will ultimately lead to advanced quality patient care.

Case Presentation 1

Leadership in Action

Pat had gone on to nursing school following graduation from high school. After spending several years working in a medical-surgical department at a large academic healthcare facility, Pat decided to obtain her APN degree. Because she had spent most of her nursing career on a medical-surgical unit providing care for patients who had undergone a surgical procedure, Pat decided that upon completion of her APN degree, she would accept a position as Clinical Specialist in the Post-Operative Recovery Unit (PACU). That way, she would be able to provide care for her surgical patients immediately following their surgical procedures. She reasoned that her understanding of how well patients recovered during their PACU experience would add tremendously to her ability to care for her patients before they were admitted to a medical-surgical unit.

Last month during the weekly healthcare team meeting, it was reported that two patients who were recently admitted to the ICU after surgery had now been confirmed with a pressure ulcer. Two weeks ago, Pat was told by the PACU internist that one patient who had recently undergone a hip replacement was diagnosed with a pressure ulcer and the patient was unable to be discharged to the rehabilitation facility. The internist also stated that the patient's hospital stay would probably be increased for several days. Last week while completing patient rounds in the PACU, Pat noticed that a patient had a reddened mark on her sacral area following cardiac surgery. Although Pat had never worked as an operating room nurse, she understood that patients should not leave the operating room with an adverse event, especially since it was not related to the surgical procedure.

With four known pressure ulcers emerging after surgery, Pat knew she must review the literature and start working on a process to minimize pressure ulcer indications on postsurgical patients.

APPLYING PATIENT QUALITY INDICATOR DATA FOR SURGICAL PRESSURE ULCERS

The critical quality indicators related to pressure ulcers (PUs) include a cadre of essential information needed to make clinical changes consistent with patient care outcomes. In order to make clinical practice changes, data associated with PUs such as severity, reimbursement for treatment, and prevention are factors associated with the outcomes from an adverse event. In this case, surgery caused the PU, thus the healthcare provider needs to know the following key points associated with PUs.

1. Pressure ulcers are defined as a localized injury to the skin and/or underlying tissue, usually over a bony prominence, as a result of pressure or pressure in combination with shear.
2. In November 2008, the Center of Medicare and Medicaid Service (CMS), started withholding payment for patients that have hospital acquired PUs (Clark 2011).
   - According to the new CMS proposal, stage three and four hospital acquired PUs outcome measures were added to the value-based incentive purchasing plan in 2014.
   - With this plan, hospitals will risk losing 1% in reimbursement if measures are not met.

3. It is estimated that intraoperative PU incidence, as a result of surgery, may be as high as 66%. Patients undergoing surgical procedures are immobile and unable to change positions, potentially increasing their risk for intraoperative PUs (Lindgren 2011).
   - The incidence among patients undergoing cardiac surgery and those with hip fractures are high.
   - Time on the operating room table, decreased circulation, and age may be predictors for PU development.
4. Implementing an aggressive preventive strategy within the operating room that would include collaboration from all perioperative areas may not only benefit patients, but may reduce costs to the healthcare facility. More clinical studies are needed to investigate the causal relationship between surgical procedures and PU development.

To assess the strategy for PU prevention for surgical patients, Pat pulled together a team of healthcare providers to decide on the quality of care framework best suited for their patient population. This team consisted of PACU, OR, Med-Surg, and Intensive Care Unit (ICU) nurses, along with two surgeons, one Internist, and one anesthesiologist. Pat knew that all healthcare personnel had to participate in developing a strategy that would be effective. Additionally, she understood that in order to implement strategic interventions for better patient outcomes, an understanding of the facility culture would be just as important. The culture of practitioners within an organization will influence any change on quality care that will be implemented. Thus, proactively engaging all healthcare providers in the problem and solution would enhance the success of any PU prevention program.

By organizing a bottoms-ups team approach, Pat was demonstrating her understanding of the normative/re-education approach (Mitchell 2013). This leadership method is based on the belief that people need to be involved or have some ownership before the practice change can be implemented. The focus is for the team to be collaborative with involvement from each member of the team, therefore, the healthcare team owns the implemented change, the process by which the change is carried out, and will be sustained to monitor the patients' outcomes.

Pat and her team chose the "Donabedian Quality of Care Framework" model. Many healthcare leaders will acknowledge that patient satisfaction is a quality indicator that has seen marked increases. However, literature is still sparse related to consensus of how patient satisfaction fits into the assessment of quality of care. The three qualities of care dimensions for measurement outlined by Donabedian are structure, process, and outcome.

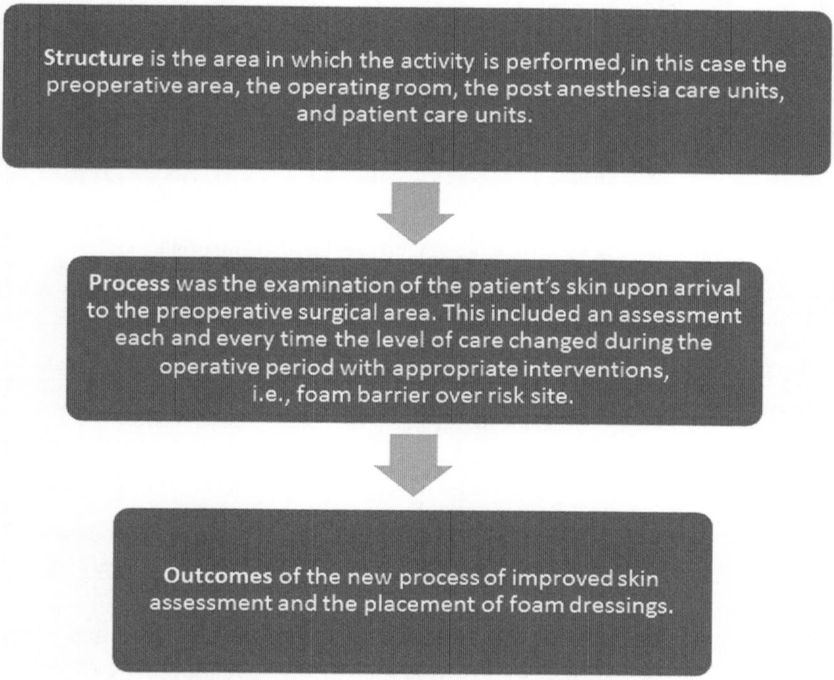

Structure is the area in which the activity is performed, in this case the preoperative area, the operating room, the post anesthesia care units, and patient care units.

Process was the examination of the patient's skin upon arrival to the preoperative surgical area. This included an assessment each and every time the level of care changed during the operative period with appropriate interventions, i.e., foam barrier over risk site.

Outcomes of the new process of improved skin assessment and the placement of foam dressings.

FIGURE 7.2. *Donabedian quality of care framework model.*

This model allows for examination of risks and hazards that exist in the structure of care that may pose a risk to patient safety, the process that defines the delivery of care, and the outcome of the interventions used to delivery patient care.

Hamrick *et al.* (2009) identified four functions characteristic of APN practice: patient care, educator, consultant, and researcher. Working in collaboration with a working healthcare team with a focus on quality patient care, Pat demonstrated her advanced leadership skills as a consultant to the team. Her advanced research on the problem of PU development during surgical procedures stood out as a key characteristic since APNs act as organizational change agents. Demonstrating her understanding of the importance of communication when providing education to the unit healthcare staff, Pat worked collaboratively with team members to provide adequate education for the practitioners who would be implementing practice changes at the bedside (Vassell *et al.* 2013).

Pat demonstrated strong leadership skills in her role as an APN in the PACU. As a result, a model of shared leadership began to emerge and a team approach formed between multiple healthcare practitioners from a variety of disciplines. The healthcare team was also provided the oppor-

TABLE 7.1. Education Interventions for Implementing a Practice Change.

Leadership in Principles	Characteristics
Education of the Staff	Intraoperative pressure ulcer development. Proper intraoperative patient positioning. How to assess for post operative pressure ulcers.
Preoperative Risk Assessment with a Tool Validated for the Operating Room	Use the assessment tool to determine individual patient interventions to protect patients from skin injuries. Assessment should become a permanent part of the chart.
Determine and Implement Protocols for Higher Risk Patients	Put in place appropriate interventions based on expert body criteria, i.e., AORN RP on patient positioning.
Effective Communication	Interprofessional communication between units and perioperative staff.
Validated Documentation to Include	What interventions did you put in place? How did you protect the patient based on the risk assessment? What was your post operative assessment immediately following surgery?

tunity to analyze the patient outcomes once the practice changes were implemented. Working collegially, the team met monthly to review actual patient cases implementing modifications to quality of care strategies. All healthcare team members were able to participate in debriefing discussions that would impact on the patient's care.

As a result of Pat's leadership and her sensitivity to being an active partner she was able to successfully provide better outcomes for the patients undergoing surgery. Additionally, she used clinical data to demonstrate effective role modeling to her colleagues. By providing clear patient centered outcomes, Pat created a successful and posi-

TABLE 7.2. Team Debrief Round Table Questions.

Question	Characteristics
1	Did working in a collaborative multidisciplinary team enhance your clinical judgment ability? If so, what new interventions were learned and implemented?
2	Do you feel the team was provided an adequate coverage of team members? If not, who would you recommend to be invited to the next meeting?
3	Did active participation from the team members change your understanding related to the culture of the facility? Based on your understanding today, would you volunteer to be a member of another facility related team?

tive strategy to promote the clinical changes necessary for effective patient care.

Case Presentation 2_____

Applying Patient Quality Indicator Data to Decrease Surgical Site Infections and Healthcare Associated Infections

Lee has been working as an APN in infection prevention for several years at a community hospital that was recently acquired by a large healthcare system. Because of the recent merging of the hospitals, physicians (including surgeons) were now given access to admit patients to the community hospital where Lee was employed. For the past year, Lee has been working with surgeons, nurses, and other healthcare providers in the OR on a preoperative patient bathing initiative as well as in the ICU implementing daily bathing for all patients.

Lee had completed her clinical research and was fully aware that preoperative patient bathing has been identified as an effective bundle strategy in the prevention of surgical site infections (SSIs) as well as hospital acquired infections (HAIs). Since HAIs and SSIs can produce high patient volumes, these infections can result in undesirable clinical outcomes such as increased length of stay and higher costs to the healthcare system.

It has been estimated that annual costs of HAI/SSI is over of $10 billion which includes both direct and indirect costs. Upon completing a thorough clinical literature review, Lee noted that the indirect cost most often seen includes the following:

- Increased pain
- Decreased quality of life
- Potential for lost wages
- Increased hospital stay

Nearly 60% of patients who acquire an SSI develop complications, often times necessitating either admission or readmission to a critical care unit. According to Bratzler and Houck (2004), readmission rates increase five-fold for those patients who acquire a SSI resulting in increased financial costs to the hospital as well as the healthcare system.

Lee was tasked with developing initiatives that would provide quality patient care in a way that the hospital would be able to quantify actual savings in infections based on strategic interventions. Working with the surgical leadership team, Lee demonstrated strong leadership skills by organizing weekly meetings addressing four primary quality indicators shown in Figure 7.3.

By implementing the four primary quality indicators, a systematic approach to developing more positive patient outcomes was initiated. Based on these quality indicators, better clinical outcomes would decrease patient infection rates, improved operational outcomes would provide clear interventions associated with preoperative bathing and critical care bathing, enhanced financial outcomes would include a decrease in SSIs or HAIs, and there would be increased cost savings based on better institutional outcomes.

During the process, Lee used Lewin's leadership style (Lewin *et al.* 1939) which included democratic leadership principles. Democratic leaders involve others in the initiative process and work with individuals to make change although they may make the final decision. Lee organized the project team, providing open communication and education on why patient bathing was so important in the fight against infections. She understood that a successful strategy to her leadership style would be to provide the staff specific examples to reach their goals.

Inherent in this leadership style is the ability to listen intently and provide examples of how to make a change. Lee decided that she needed to implement the clinical changes needed during different phases of the patients care both prior and during the patient's hospitalization.

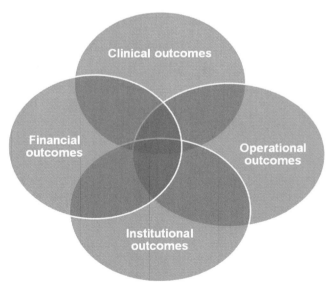

FIGURE 7.3. Adapted from the Battie-Dopp Model using outcome indicators of the SCIP model.

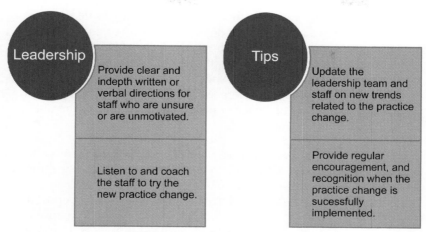

FIGURE 7.4. Leadership coaching tips.

1. Phase one of the initiative for patient bathing was implemented in the ICU with much success. Staff, patients, and families were all given education on the reasons patient bathing was important to enhance the patient's quality of care and enhance their outcomes while in the hospital.

2. In phase two, preoperative bathing prior to surgery was also implemented for all surgical patients. Lee created specific organizational protocols that would be utilized at both the hospital and the surgeon's offices. Over 90% of all surgical groups readily accepted the new bathing guidelines for their patients. However, because of the merger of this facility within a larger healthcare system, Lee had encountered some push back or noncompliance from several surgical groups who did not support the principles associated with patient bathing.

Based on her knowledge of the Institute of Medicine's description of the six steps for high patient quality care (IOM 2001), Lee decided to review the characteristics of each step prior to meeting individually with those surgeons who were unsure of the goals of the patient bathing initiative.

By discussing the importance of bathing through the use of the patient safety framework from IOM, Lee was able to provide data to surgeons about the need to change their current thinking about the principles of presurgical bathing.

3. Lastly, a change of culture from one healthcare facility to another

can be extremely slow to adopt any practice changes. Healthcare disciplines have always relied on their own way of doing things within their culture and subcultures, that is, nurses, physicians, anesthesiologists, and other healthcare providers. These subcultures are defined by their own specificity, practices, or ethics. Lee demonstrated strong leadership skills by her understanding that due to the diversity of varied cultures, practice changes are not simple and they are not quick.

Being aware that even the most well-planned patient quality initiatives can ultimately fail if those within the organization do not embrace the current culture was important for Lee's ultimate success.

Lee recognized that she would need to take on the role of consultant when meeting with the surgeons in order to achieve high quality care for all patients within the accepted standardized protocols. In essence, Lee was also assuming the role of a change agent. By doing so, she was able to network with other leaders and/or change agents within the healthcare system eliciting support for the practice change. Based on Lewin's (1974) second stage of change, which involves transition to the

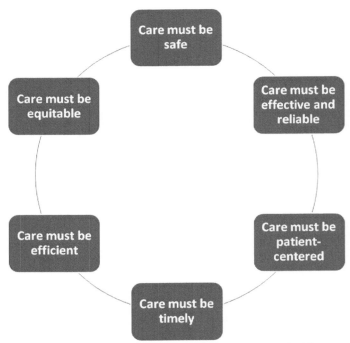

FIGURE 7.5. Institute of Medicine's six steps to high quality healthcare.

desired state, Lee identified strategies where supporters and opponents of the practice change were identified. Being a change agent for the process, Lee was able to strengthen the initiative, while encouraging multidirectional communication between all parties, informing the surgeons of the exact practice change which provided them and their office staff essential content and written material. Lee practiced strong negotiation skills when she met with the surgeon opponents by providing them evidence-based practice documents to support the patient bathing initiative as a patient quality care initiative.

Ensuring quality nursing care is the cornerstone in the delivery of positive patient outcomes. In a study by Kalisch (2006), RNs, LPNs, and NAs were interviewed in multiple focus groups. All of the focus group participants stated that they did not or were not able to provide all of the nursing care that their patients needed. Areas of missed care included ambulation, turning, delayed feedings, patient education, discharge planning, hygiene, and surveillance. The participant's reasons for the missed patient care included time, too few staff, poor use of resources, habit, denial, and ineffective delegation. The results of this study as well as like studies provide further validation that APNs are required more today than in past years thus confirming the need for more APNs as we move in healthcare of the future.

APNs are taking their place in the forefront of today's rapidly changing healthcare system, by developing a myriad of roles within the organization with a goal to augment cost-effective, quality patient care (Jansen 2010). APNs must be grounded in theory and research to guide to their clinical practice. They must feel confident and competent to work in collegial relationships with physicians, nurses, and other multidisciplinary healthcare providers. These roles and responsibilities require APNs who are well educated yet caring and compassionate professionals.

SUMMARY POINTS

- In order to implement high patient quality outcomes, APNs must recognize that change is expected and essential for the growth that is needed to understand new trending.
- As leaders within the hospital, APNs are expected to provide insight for new clinical practice initiatives that will promote positive patient outcomes.
- APNs are expected to work collaboratively and collegially with other disciplines within the healthcare facility.
- APNs must embrace the cultural diversity of the healthcare facility as well as the practitioners who deliver patient care.

- APNs should provide clarity for evidence-based practice and the ongoing changes to those within the facility as appropriate.
- APNs take on multiple roles that include, consultant, educator, process leader, etc., based on the current initiative.

REFERENCES

Bratzler, D.W. and P.M. Houck. 2004. Antimicrobial prophylaxis for surgery: An advisory statement from the National Surgical Infection Prevention Project. *Clin Infect Dis; 38* (1706–15).

Clark, C. 2011. CMS releases value-based purchasing incentive plan. *Health Leaders Media.* Accessed November, 2013. http://www.healthleadersmedia.com/page-3/HEP-261211/CMS-Releases-ValueBased-Purchasing-Incentive-Plan

Hamric, A., J. Spross, and C. Hanson. 2009. *Advanced practice nursing: An integrative approach.* Philadelphia: Elsevier.

Ibn, H., M. Lamrini, and N. Rais. 2006. Donabedian Model (Committee on Redesigning Health Insurance Performance Measures, Payment, and Performance Improvement Programs).

Institute of Medicine (IOM). 2001. *Crossing the Quality Chasm: A New Health System for the 21st Century.* Committee on Quality of Health Care in America, of Medicine. Washington, DC. National Academies Press.

Jansen, M. and M. Zwygart-Stauffacher. 2010. *Advanced Practice Nursing Core Concepts for Professional Role Development.* Springer Publishing Company, LLC, NY.

Kalisch, B. 2006. Missed Nursing Care; A Qualitative Study. *J Nurs Care Qual.* Vol. 21, No. 4, (306–313). Lippincott Williams & Wilkins Inc.

Lewin, K., R. Lippit, and R. White. 1939. Patterns of aggressive behavior in experimentally created social climates. *Journal of Social Psychology, 10*, (271–301).

Lindgren, M., M. Unosson, A.M. Krantz, and C. Eka. 2005. Pressure ulcer risk factors in patients undergoing surgery. *Journal of Advanced Nursing 50*(6) (605–612).

Mitchell, G. 2013. Selecting the best theory to implement planned change. *Nursing Management 20*, (1) (32–37).

Vassell, P., D. Fawcett, and J. Seltzer. 2013. *Emerging Trends: Pressure Ulcer Prevention in the Operating Room.* OR Manager Conference, October 2013.

World Health Organization (WHO). 2006. Quality of care: a process for making strategic choices in health systems (4).

Principles of Quality and Safe Patient Care

MARY E. ASHER DNP, RN, CNS, CPAN

Chapter 8 discusses the principles associated with quality and safe patient care. A case study about the prevention of medical errors associated with patient safety is presented and discussed.

Case Presentation

In 1976, Mr. Hennessy, a 60% disabled veteran, had his first open heart surgery. He had a 90% occlusion of the right anterior descending artery which required open heart surgery for a triple bypass in a major military hospital. Eight hours after surgery when he was extubated, his chest tubes filled with blood. He was awake and alert as he was rolled into the OR with the surgeon's hand in his thoracic cavity holding pressure on the "bleed." Because of hemorrhaging, he received numerous emergency blood transfusions. Unfortunately, this would come back to haunt him 30 years later when, at the age of 80, he was diagnosed with Hepatitis C.

The surgeon came out to talk with his wife. He spoke calmly as he tried to assure her that Mr. Hennessy was doing well. He was extremely surprised when Mr. Hennessy's wife stated, "Don't talk down to me. You screwed up or we would not be here right now. Be honest and tell me exactly what happened and how are you going to handle my husband's situation?" The surgeon took a deep breath and then began to explain the entire situation.

Mr. Hennessy's health was stable for the next 22 years. In 1998, Mr. Hennessy was admitted to the hospital with severe chest pain and required open heart surgery in 3 days once he was stabilized. He was scheduled for a triple bypass graft and aortic valve replacement.

Mr. Hennessy's wife and daughter sat in the waiting room while he had surgery. As they waited, they became aware of several other family members waiting for their loved ones. They had a conversation with a very pleasant middle-aged man. He told them the reason his mother was in the OR was because "they had left sponges in her abdomen." Evidently, his mother had had abdominal surgery about 7 days before, and after surgery kept complaining of abdominal symptoms. The attending found on x-ray that there were at least two gauze sponges left in her abdomen.

Imagine the family's concern; the last thing a family member wants to hear is that there was an OR error when their "loved one" is in the OR. This experience questioned the quality and safety of the hospital and healthcare personnel. Since the daughter was a nurse, she reassured Mr. Hennessy's wife that his sponge count would be correct; every nurse in the hospital's OR that day would be aware an error had been made so they would be extremely cautious on their sponge counts. Fortunately, Mr. Hennessy came though his surgery with flying colors.

Following his surgery, Mr. Hennessy developed a pleural effusion which made it difficult to sleep well at night. He always had extremely sensitive hearing and the noise of the ICU drove him crazy. After 3 days, he was released to the telemetry unit to a private room.

On the fourth day after his second open heart surgery, at 3:30 A.M. Mr. Hennessy's daughter went to the hospital because the nurse phoned the family about Mr. Hennessy's sleeplessness. When his daughter arrived at the hospital she spoke directly to the young night nurse to see what needed to be done. All Mr. Hennessy wanted was to sleep. Activities were clustered: EKG, CXR, pain medication, and drawing labs from the central line. Mr. Hennessy was then repositioned, his head elevated, and he fell asleep immediately. His daughter spent the next four nights at Mr. Hennessy's bedside to promote his rest and sleep.

In 2005, Mr. Hennessy began experiencing severe fatigue. Initially, no one thought much of it because of his cardiac history; however, eventually he was diagnosed with Hepatitis C. The only risk factor he had was the emergency blood transfusions he had during surgery back in 1976. Mr. Hennessy was not given any aggressive treatment for the disease; however, he had sporadic episodes of fatigue and then weeks of feeling better.

In March 2012, Mr. Hennessy, then 85 years old, was admitted to the hospital for a fractured hip. He went for surgery 3 days later, had spinal anesthesia, and came through the surgery well. On the third day postop he began having severe postoperative complications. His BUN and creatinine levels became elevated and he developed anasarca, severe swelling in the abdominal/pelvic area.

Mr. Hennessy remained in this community hospital for the next 16 days trying to improve enough to go to the acute rehabilitation hospital. Unfortunately, the quality of the nursing care in this hospital was extremely variable. Some days the care was good, other days the care was marginal. Mr. Hennessy finally improved physically enough to be transferred to the acute rehabilitation hospital.

Mr. Hennessy was placed in the acute rehabilitation hospital for 4 weeks. The hospital care was truly interdisciplinary. The physicians made rounds with the nurses and they had a very collaborative approach to patient care. At the end of the 4 weeks his hip had healed. Thus, he transferred to the rehabilitation hospital near his house by ambulance.

After 3 days in the rehabilitation hospital, Mr. Hennessy became weak and very tired. All he wanted was to sleep. His condition became worse and it was determined he would not make it back to his home after his time in rehabilitation. A discussion was held with his daughter (his healthcare surrogate and advocate) about placing him in hospice care. Laboratory tests demonstrated a WBC count of 19,000 which indicated sepsis. The decision was made not to readmit him to the hospital that afternoon. That evening at 9 P.M., Mr. Hennessy died peacefully, surrounded by loved ones.

QUALITY AND SAFETY ISSUES IN HEALTHCARE

In 1976, Mr. Hennessy, a 60% disabled veteran, had his first open heart surgery. At that time he had a 90% occlusion of his right anterior ascending artery. He ended up having open heart surgery for a triple bypass in a major military hospital.

The above case presentation demonstrates that obtaining quality and safe healthcare in today's healthcare environment remains challenging. With an aging, increasingly diverse population and rapidly changing healthcare system, trying to provide quality healthcare to Americans will continue to be a major challenge. According to the Institute of Medicine (2011), APNs must be prepared to participate to the "full extent of their education and training" in order for Americans to receive high quality and safe healthcare in the future. Nurses must be actively engaged in their profession and be lifelong learners in order to have the skills needed to succeed in the rapidly changing healthcare environment of the United States.

During Mr. Hennessy's second open heart surgery in 1998, his wife and daughter sat in the waiting room. While waiting, they became aware of other families. They had a conversation with a pleasant middle-aged man. He told them the reason his mother was in the OR was because "they had left sponges in her abdomen." His mother had abdominal surgery 7 days before, and after surgery kept complaining of abdominal symptoms. X-rays confirmed there were two gauze sponges left in her abdomen.

For the past decade, the prevention of medical errors and promotion of patient safety within the American healthcare system has been a major initiative. Within the United States, safety is a fundamental core value in the healthcare environment of which nursing is an integral member. They are the largest group of healthcare providers within the hospital setting, and nurses have a moral and legal obligation to protect their patients from harm. Most often they are the direct care givers and the last line of defense in preventing medical errors and patient safety issues.

Imagine Mr. Hennessy's family's concern during his second open heart surgery; the last thing they needed to hear was about the error in the OR. This experience questioned the quality and safety of the hospital and healthcare personnel. Mr. Hennessy's daughter was a nurse and she reassured Mrs. Hennessy the sponge count would be correct; every nurse in the hospital's OR that day would be aware of the error which had been made.

To Err is Human: Building a Safer Health Care System was the catalyst to force major change within the American healthcare system to promote quality patient care and safe patient outcomes (IOM 1999). As many as 98,000 people die each year from medical errors that occur in hospitals (IOM 1999). In response to specific problems of safety within the American healthcare environment, the Joint Commission in 2003 developed the National Patient Safety Goals. Each year these goals are updated and can be viewed online (Joint Commission 2014).

In 2003, the National Research Council issued a report entitled *Health Professions Education: A Bridge to Quality*. The outcome of this report was the delineation of essential required core knowledge which should be included in all healthcare professions education. These areas of core knowledge emphasized patient-centered care, interdisciplinary teams, evidenced-based practice, quality improvement, and informatics (The National Research Council 2003). Furthermore, the report *The Future of Nursing Leading Change, Advancing Health* (IOM 2011) advocated for profound changes to the education and training system for both undergraduate and graduate nurses in order to provide the work force needed for the future. "Nursing education at all levels needs to provide a better understanding of and experience with case management, quality improvement methods, systems-level change management, and the reconceptualized roles of nurses in a reformed healthcare system," (IOM 2011).

In response to the IOM reports, the Robert Wood Johnson Foundation funded the Quality and Safety Education for Nurses (QSEN) initiative in 2005. The major leaders of the project were Dr. Linda Cronenwett and Dr. Gwen Sherwood at the School of Nursing of the University of North Carolina at Chapel Hill. The purpose of the QSEN initiative was to address the issue of preparing future nurses with the necessary competencies needed to improve the quality and safety of the healthcare systems in which they worked (Cronenwett *et al.* 2007). According to Sullivan, the QSEN initiative was created to "produce graduates who based their practice on a spirit of inquiry and continuous improvement, who would ask questions about what and how they delivered care and how patient outcomes are monitored (2009). The QSEN reviewed the IOM reports and accepted the five core knowledge areas: (1) patient-centered care, (2) teamwork and collaboration, (3) evidenced based practice, (4) quality improvement, and (5) informatics as important to nursing practice. However, the QSEN went on to include safety as a needed sixth core knowledge area for nursing practice (QSEN Institute 2014).

Embedded within each competency are specific skills, knowledge, and attitudes. The competencies are for both prelicensure and graduate level nursing education. Examples of integrating quality and safety content which are evidence-based into clinical teaching are now just appearing in the literature. Clinical faculty need to start shifting from an individual focus to a systems focus in acute care. Premeim *et al.* (2009) suggests ways to begin implementing the six QSEN competencies into the fundamentals of nursing education. Faculty of graduate nursing programs have also examined their curricula to include the six QSEN competencies. All aspects of the curriculum have been included in the review, specifically the lectures, clinical simulations, and other clinical learning assignments. Premeim *et al.* states, "The QSEN framework provides a useful organizing scheme, competency definitions, and relevant associations between basic nursing care and contemporary quality and safety national initiatives" (2009).

On the fourth day after his second open heart surgery, the nurse telephoned the family at 2 A.M. regarding Mr. Hennessy's sleeplessness. When his daughter arrived at the hospital, she spoke directly to the young night nurse to see what needed to be done.

All Mr. Hennessy wanted was to sleep. Activities were clustered: EKG, CXR, pain medication, and drawing labs from the central line. Mr. Hennessy was then repositioned, his head elevated, and he fell asleep immediately. His daughter spent the next four nights at Mr. Hennessy's bedside to promote his rest and sleep.

Being a competent nurse caring for diverse populations across the lifespan requires lifelong learning. Continuing education hours are required by many states to renew nursing licensure. However, this is an external motivator for nurses. Being a lifelong learner requires an individual to be internally motivated. Nurses who want to provide quality and safe patient care will be internally driven and will be motivated to keep pace with the latest in research. The next generation of nurses will be required to develop a spirit of inquiry, will value lifelong education, and will use informatics to deliver quality care based on the "evidence" (Benner *et al.* 2010).

THE ROLE OF THE ADVANCED PRACTICE NURSE IN PROMOTING QUALITY/SAFE CARE

The roles of the APN are numerous and varied across the United States; as the American healthcare system advances and changes, so will the roles of advanced practice nurses. Currently, the roles of the advanced practice nurse in the clinical setting include nurse practitioners (NPs), certified registered nurse anesthetists (CRNAs), clinical nurse specialists (CNSs), and certified nurse midwives (CNMs) (IOM 2011). Academic roles include the nurse researcher and nurse educator. The final role is the nurse leader which is found in the political arena, the academic setting, and in large healthcare systems. In the future, these roles will impact the quality and safety of patient care in both rural and large metropolitan healthcare settings.

Education Roles

Academic partnerships have been identified as the foundation on which to transform nursing education in American in order to meet the needs of a modern workforce (Benner *et al.* 2010). Nursing researchers' primary focus is to advance nursing science and knowledge. Expanded collaboration between academic health science centers and healthcare systems are on the upswing. Joint positions are being developed between hospital systems and academics whereby nursing researchers and educators promote research and evidence-based nursing practice. The work load for these advance practice nurses are split between the university and the hospital system. Advance practice nurses serve as a bridge between the "ivory tower and the real world." Having strong communication between academic and healthcare systems promotes an understanding of the issues encountered within the complex American health system. Collaboration between the newly developed role of the Doctorate in Nursing Practice (DNP) and the existing nursing scientist role (PhD) should result in increased nursing research and knowledge. Together, these advanced practice nurses can help develop nursing science and promote the development of a modern nursing work force.

> Mr. Hennessy was placed in the acute rehabilitation hospital for four weeks. The medical and nursing care was good overall, and Mr. Hennessy slowly improved. The hospital care was truly interdisciplinary. The physicians made rounds with the nurses and they had a very collaborative approach to patient care.

Interdisciplinary education has been determined to be critical for developing a well trained work force. According to Benner *et al.*, "Nursing, medicine, physical therapy, and other healthcare professionals educate their students in academic silos, isolated from one another and hence largely ignorant of the expertise of those with whom they will need to work closely and seamlessly," (2010). The focus of education for nurses in the future requires the use of simulation and web-based learning. These two methods of education can easily be incorporated into interprofessional education. Simulation allows students to "make mistakes" in a safe learning environment. A major attribute to web-based learning is the flexibility of scheduling instruction for numerous students. If nursing students can be educated in aspects of interpersonal collaboration with other health professional students through simulation and web-based learning, upon graduation these students should be able to work more collaboratively with other disciplines (IOM 2011c).

Clinical Practice Roles

By the year 2015, nurses seeking to become ANPs will be required to have a doctorate in nursing practice (DNP) in order to be licensed (AACN 2014). As a result of the NP movement, NPs are now employed in both the primary care and acute care setting in urban and rural areas. The expansion of the scope of practice for NPs has allowed access to quality and safe healthcare to patients who otherwise would not have a healthcare provider available. Due to the shortages of primary care providers and the increase in the numbers of patients who now can access health insurance, NPs continue to provide healthcare services in frontier, rural, and underserved areas of the United States (IOM 2011e).

Under the Affordable Care Act, nurse managed clinics will be expanded and APNs will work within multidisciplinary teams to provide comprehensive health services. Due to an aging population of patients with chronic illnesses, the demand for health services will increase in an already overloaded healthcare system. NPs are uniquely positioned to meet the challenge of the elderly patient with chronic illness (Watts *et al.* 2009). In a qualitative case analysis, Watts *et al.* (2009) found that nurse practitioners are very effective in group visits or shared medical appointments (SMAs), especially in a chronic care model (CCM). The three areas NPs had the greatest impact was self-management, decision support, and delivery design. The study demonstrated that when nurses are allowed to practice to the fullest extent of their education and training, patients have better outcomes. According to the American Association of Colleges of Nursing (AACN), quality/safe patient care is enhanced by having a well-educated nursing workforce (2014). When nurses have higher levels of education, there are lower mortality rates, more positive outcomes for patients, and less medication errors (AACN 2014).

With the Affordable Care Act, new opportunities will present themselves for APNs. Current models of care which have been developed include the Accountable Care Organizations (ACOs), Medical/Health Homes, Community Health Centers (CHCs), and Nurse-Managed Health Centers (NMHCs). Other healthcare models may not have yet been developed. According to the IOM (2011), nurses need to collaborate with other professionals to create innovative care delivery models which provide quality, safe, and cost-effective care. Innovative solutions are possible when nursing researchers work in partnership with other professionals such as business, law, medicine, and technology.

Leadership Roles

All nurses from the bedside to the boardroom will need strong leadership skills to deal with the challenges facing the modern healthcare system in America. Nursing leaders will need to apply the concepts of complex system science to the traditional management concepts of planning, organizing, directing, coordinating, and controlling patient care. They will need to embrace technology as a key tool for developing computational models and simulation for nursing research within their institutions. Nursing leaders will need to support nursing informatics to further nursing practice, research, and education within the American healthcare system (Clancy *et al.* 2008).

Strong leadership skills are necessary for all nurses working within complex health systems. Patient advocacy is a primary role for nursing. Nurses can and should advocate at the bedside or in the home (the micro system); they can and should advocate for quality and safe patient care as chief nursing officers (CNOs) or as members of health policy committees (the macro system). Nursing leaders need to possess the ability to work as members of teams, be knowledgeable of patient care delivery systems, and be able to collaborate across and within disciplines (IOM 2011). All nurses must recognize that strong leadership skills are as important as strong clinical skills when promoting quality and safe patient care.

The role of APNs is to serve as leaders in promoting quality/safe patient care in the hospital and community settings and at the local, state, and national level. Nurses can no longer "sit in the back seat," but must seek to be in "the driver's seat" in promoting quality outcomes for individual patients and communities. There are currently over 3.1 million licensed registered nurses (RNs) in the United States (American Nurses Association 2011). If all RNs were politically involved, nursing would have enormous power in the political system within the United States. The current number of RNs prepared as APNs is only 250,527, which accounts for approximately 8% of the RN workforce in America. Sixty percent of nursing faculty is over the age of 50, and the average age of RNs is currently 45.5 years of age. Therefore, there is a great need for developing a larger work force that increases and an increased number of APNs and nursing faculty within the next 10 years (American Nurses Association 2011).

APNS must lead the charge in promoting nursing as a valued profession. All APNs in their various roles serve as role models for both the public and the nursing profession. Mentoring nursing students and younger nurses is part of lifelong learning and "all nurses have the responsibility to mentor those who come after them," (IOM 2011). Furthermore, one of the greatest needs in nursing is to have APNs involved in policy making. This involvement can be on the local level such as school boards, or by running for political office on the local, state, or even national level. These positions require APNs to have strong communication skills, networking skills, and political savvy. APNS serving in a political office will help promote quality, safe, and affordable healthcare.

Promoting safe and quality patient care is an integral part of the APN's role. Having insight into systems theory and complex systems theories enables APNs to begin to resolve issues/problems and design plans of care to promote quality outcomes. Nurses work in a complex world with complicated problems. All APNs, regardless of their roles, need to be actively involved when problem solving in their healthcare organizations. Through communication, collaboration, research, and evidence-based practice APNs are uniquely qualified to promote quality, safe, and cost-effective care in the new American healthcare system.

SUMMARY POINTS

- Nurses are the direct care givers and the last line of defense in preventing medical errors and patient safety issues.
- Nursing education must promote the QSEN core competencies for both undergraduate and graduate nursing programs: patient-centered care, interdisciplinary teams, evidence-based practice, quality improvement, informatics, and safety.
- Collaboration between the DNP and the PhD should result in increased nursing research and knowledge.
- Advocacy is a primary role for all nurses and APNs to promote quality, safe, and cost-effective care.
- Leadership must be practiced by all nurses and APNS from the bedside to the board room to promote quality, safe, and cost-effective outcomes.

REFERENCES

American Association of Colleges of Nursing. 2014a. *Creating a more highly qualified nursing workforce.* Retrieved March 19, 2014. http://www.aacn.nche.edu/media-relations/fact-sheets/nursing-workforce

American Association of Colleges of Nursing. 2014b. *Doctor of nursing practice.* Retrieved March 18, 2014. http://www.aacn.nche.edu/dnp

American Nurses Association. 2011. *American nurses association fact sheet.* Retrieved March 20, 2014.http://nursingworld.org/NursingbytheNumbersFactSheet

Benner, P., M. Stuphen, V. Leonard, and L. Day. 2010. *Educating Nurses: A call for radical reform.* San Francisco, CA: Jossey-Bass.

Chaffee, M.W. and M.M. McNeill. 2007. A model of nursing as a complex adaptive system. *Nursing Outlook, 55,* 232–241. doi:10.1016/j.outlook.2007.04.003

Clancy, T.R., J.A. Effken, and D. Pesut. 2008. Applications of complex systems theory in nursing education research and practice. *Nursing Outlook, 56*(5), 248. doi:10.1016/j.outlook.2008.06.010

Cronenwett, L., G. Sherwood, J. Barnsteiner, J. Disch, P. Jonson, P. Mitchel,P., 1 D. Sullivan, J. Warren. 2007. Quality and safety education for nurses. *Nursing Outlook, 55*(3), 121–131. doi:10.1016/j.outlook.2007.02.006

Institute of Medicine. 1999. *To err is human: Building a safer health system.* Retrieved March 18, 2014. http://http://www.iom.edu/~/media/Files/Report%20Files/1999/To-Err-is-Human/To%20Err%20is%20Human%201999%20%20report%20brief.pdf

Institute of Medicine 2011a. Transforming Leadership. In *The future of nursing leading change, advancing health* (244). Washington, DC: Institute of Medicine of the National Academies.

Institute of Medicine. 2011b. The future of nursing: Leading change, advancing health. Washington, DC: The National Academies Press.

Institute of Medicine. 2011c. Transforming Education. In *The future of nursing leading change, advancing health* (163–219). Washington, DC: Institute of Medicine of the National Academies.

Institute of Medicine. 2011d. Transforming Practice. In *The future of nursing leading change, advancing health* (85–162). Washington, DC: Institute of Medicine of the National Academies.

Institute of Medicine. 2011e. Key messages of the report. In *The future of nursing leading change, advancing health* (21–45). Washington, DC: Institute of Medicine of the National Academies.

Joint Commission. 2013. *National Patient Safety Goals Effective January 1, 2014.* Retrieved March 21, 2014. http://www.jointcommission.org/assets/1/6/HAP_NPSG_Chapter_2014.pdf

Joint Commission. 2014. 2014 *National patient safety goals slide presentation.* Retrieved March 19, 2014. http://http://www.jointcommission.org/standards_information/npsgs.aspx

The National Research Council. 2003. *Health professions education: A bridge to quality.* Retrieved March 20, 2014. http://www.nap.edu/catalog.php?record_id=10681

Premeim, G., G.E. Armstrong, and A.J. Barton. 2009. The new fundamentals in nursing: Introducing beginning quality and safety education for nurses' competencies. *Journal of Nursing Education, 48*(12), 694-697. doi:10.3928/01484834-20091113-10

QSEN Institute. 2005–2014. *Competencies.* Retrieved March 18, 2014. http://qsen.org/competencies

Sullivan, D. 2009. Quality and Safety education for nurses: A National Initiative funded by the Robert Wood Johnson Foundation. *Creative Nursing, 15* (2), 111. doi:10.1891/1078-4535.15.2.111

Watts, S.A., J. Gee, M.E. O'Day, K. Schaub, R. Lawrence, and D. Aron, *et al.* 2009. Nurse practitioner-led multidisciplinary teams to improve chronic illness care: the unique strengths of nurse practitioners applied to shared medical appointments/group visits. *Journal of the American Academy of Nurse Practioners, 21* (167–172). doi:10.1111/j.1745-7599.2008.00379

Understanding the Role of Leadership and Critical Thinking Principles to Improve Patient Outcomes

MARY M. WYCKOFF PHD., NNP-BC, ACNP, BC, FNP-BC, CCNS, CCRN, FAANP

Chapter 9 includes a case study that demonstrates the role of leadership and critical thinking principles that are associated with systems approaches, which accelerate improving patient outcomes. These approaches further analyze error prevention, debriefing, and organizational communication.

Case Presentation

Ashley Mason is a PHD. registered nurse leader who is the system manager of a 600 bed university teaching facility, which provides healthcare to a large, inner city population of patients. This population has had difficulty accessing healthcare, and primary preventative care has not always been readily accessible. Many of the situations which arise are urgent and emergent requiring astute leadership skills to manage difficult circumstances. Ashley has developed the vision of a transformational leader which encompasses a vision of the future that will excite and begin a broad series of discussions of how to shape the future success of team concepts (Bass 1990, 1985). Becoming a transformational leader involves being an emissary and visionary of where we are now and where we want to go. Having individuals buy into this team concept is the key to successful transformational leadership and becoming the efficacious leader necessary to move institutional change forward (Northouse 2012).

The emergency medical system (EMS) has advised the emergency department (ED) that a 32-year-old female of unknown gestational age without prenatal care has been involved in a motor vehicle crash and is in acute distress secondary to chest pain and abdominal pain. The ED system alert is activated to notify the ED staff and trauma team which includes an anesthesiologist, obstetrics (OB) team, and neonatal intensive care (NICU) team.

The patient arrives within 4 minutes of notification and teams are assembled within the trauma area awaiting notification of need. The trauma and OB teams' predetermined leaders examine the patient while fetal heart tones are being evaluated. The initial 1-minute assessment leads to concerns that the patient is abrupting her placenta and the infant is in danger from placental hemorrhage. The fetal heart tones over the next minute are determined to be non-reassuring. The viability of the infant is determined based upon the emergent ultrasound and size of the uterus. The trauma team and OB teams are prepared to facilitate an emergency cesarean section and stabilize her trauma needs, including maintaining her spinal immobilization, intubation, and sustainability of life. Emergency subclavian lines are placed by the trauma resident while the OB team chief resident prepares for emergent delivery. The NICU team is prepared for an emergent delivery of an estimated 29–30 week infant with a full resuscitation prepared, including intubation, umbilical catheterization, volume resuscitation, and emergency medications for full resuscitation.

Within 3 minutes of arrival, the infant is delivered. Every team manages their own individual entity. The mother was managed for all traumatic injury, chest and abdomen with combined efforts of hemorrhage control by OB and trauma, and the infant was managed by the NICU team. The infant was estimated at less than 900 grams requiring intubation secondary to failed 30 seconds of continuous positive airway pressure (CPAP) while being dried and wrapped in plastic wrap for warmth, including a congruent assessment of a heart rate less than 60 beats per minute requiring compressions. An umbilical catheter was placed and volume resuscitation of 20 ml/kg normal saline was infused. The Apgar's were 1, 5, and 7 and the infant was transported to the NICU in a heated isolette.

The mother was stabilized and was able to have scans to assess her for further injury. Her assessment showed a fractured right knee and right pelvic rami fracture requiring stabilization. The mother was transported post operatively to the trauma intensive care unit.

Ashley Mason is the leader responsible for the quality and management of system responsiveness to urgent and emergent situations and analyzes the outcomes and functions of the teams. This required massive organization and coordination for one trauma patient that subsequently becomes two and requires interdisciplinary coordination of not only system management, but also team and individual management. In order to achieve these functional goals there are detailed concepts that must be put into place to achieve successful outcomes, and everyone must know their role to function independently and interdependently while still functioning interdisciplinary (AHRQ 2008; Baker *et al.* 2005).

ESSENTIAL PRINCIPLES FOR SUCCESSFUL TEAMS

Ashley is very aware that the only way a situation as described above can lead to successful outcomes is through by a systematic and organized team. The success of this situation can only be achieved through coordination of multiple teams, strong communication, leadership, successful dynamics, and practice sessions such as drills incorporating simulation to prepare for response teams to complex, high-risk circumstances. Ashley utilized the TeamSTEPPS® program, which was developed by the Department of Defense (DoD) patient safety program to in collaboration with the Agency for Healthcare Research and Quality (AHRQ 2012, 2008) (Figure 9.1).

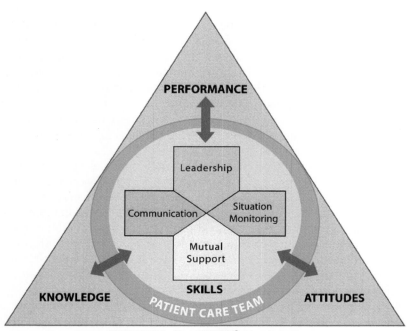

FIGURE 9.1. *TeamSTEPPS® triangle logo.*

TeamSTEPPS®

The TeamSTEPPS® triangle logo is a visual model that represents some basic but critical concepts related to teamwork training. Individuals can learn four primary trainable teamwork skills:

1. Leadership
2. Communication
3. Situation monitoring
4. Mutual support

If a team has tools and strategies, it can leverage to build a fundamental level of competency in each of those skills. Research has shown that the team can enhance three types of teamwork outcomes:

1. Performance
2. Knowledge
3. Attitudes

For example, if every member of the team has basic competency in situation monitoring and communication, it is incumbent upon them to build shared mental models more effectively. Improved outcomes beget greater proficiency (improved teamwork skills) and a desire to be a part of the team (attitudes). Such is the reciprocal relationship between skills and outcomes. The systematic goal is to facilitate the development of high-quality team management and to minimize the human factors, which are inherent to error. There are human limitations related to each clinical case or situation that requires detailed communications, individual back up, and support that will reduce secondary sequelae (Kohn *et al.* 2000). Incorporating these skills with team management, leadership skills, prebriefing, and debriefing will provide enhanced safety and decrease human error.

Most healthcare professionals do not enter healthcare systems with team education or training since most health professional curricula has been offered through advanced educational programs (Awad *et al.* 2005). However, facility quality reviews and team coordination is a substantial part of the organizational structure of the leadership team. These dynamics need to be organized and developed prior to the situational occurrence (Mann *et al.* 2006). Often, essential content related to team building has been minimally provided thus leaving room for continuing education related to effective team management.

In 1999, preventable medical errors in United States hospitals were estimated to cost $17–$29 billion dollars and the morbidity of patients was estimated to be 98,000 patient lives annually (Kohn *et al.* 2000).

These errors are reducible by instituting strong leadership skills, team development, and coordination of care teams, and by providing a cadre of team training modules that enhance team building across disciplines (AHRQ 2012).

> Ashley, as the leader of this inner city healthcare facility, coordinated meetings to facilitate the intercommunication between multiple teams. The development of these teams was built on communication and leadership knowledge.

Leaders must have an identified knowledge base, skill, and the ability to function in stressful situations, while analyzing complex human factors and behaviors. High performing team leaders and members must share a clear vision of the plan by utilizing structured communication, adapting to rapid or unstable situations, and working across disciplines. If all members of the interdisciplinary healthcare team work toward the same goal, optimal patient safety outcomes can be achieved (AHRQ 2008).

Essential Team Competencies

Teamwork competencies include strong leadership skills that involve the ability to direct and coordinate team members, assign roles, motivate team members, and facilitate optimal team performance. The leader further needs to be able to clarify team roles, provide performance expectations, facilitate prebriefing, team problem solving, and debriefing discussions (AHRQ 2012).

> The ED system alert is activated to notify the ED staff and trauma team, which includes an anesthesiologist, OB team, and NICU team.
> The patient arrives within 4 minutes of notification and teams are assembled within the trauma area awaiting notification of need. The trauma and OB teams' predetermined leaders examine the patient while fetal heart tones are being evaluated. The initial 1-minute assessment leads to concerns that the patient is abrupting her placenta and the infant is in danger from placental hemorrhage.

In the case scenario, the activation of teams is predetermined based on the information received. When EMS notified the ED team of their situation, the ED leader, who is usually the nurse in charge, activated the notification system of the teams. In this situation, it involved three essential groups: anesthesia, the trauma team, the OB emergency team, and the NICU team.

Facilitating Teams

The coordination of each individual team is the responsibility of the team leader who coordinates with leaders of the other specialty teams. These teams are not only multidisciplinary but also interdisciplinary. The teams include professionals from nursing, technicians, chaplains, pharmacists, physicians, residents, fellows, nurse practitioners, physician assistants, environmental specialists, electronic medical record facilitators, and many other members who facilitate the function of the facility. In this case scenario, over 25 team members were present, which, if not coordinated properly, could have easily turned into a chaotic situation. For example, if the noise level in the room was loud, it would have been difficult to communicate and the teams would have been disorganized. Unfortunately, disorganized teams lead to unsuccessful patient outcomes. If the communication is clear, concise, and organized, team members are able to repeat the communication, and then the functioning of the team is effective (Haig *et al.* 2006; Pronovost *et al.* 2003).

Principles of Prebriefing

Prebriefing facilitates determination of who is responsible for each situation. Delineation of roles needs to be predetermined. For example, the trauma team leader will be the trauma fellow, and his back up will be the trauma attending, and the roles are then assigned. The anesthesia resident will manage the airway, the chief will be back up, the second trauma resident and trauma nurse will manage cervical spine and back, while the trauma physician assistant will place the subclavian line. The OB team chief, whose back up is the third year resident, will facilitate the ultrasound while the OB nurse manages the fetal monitoring. The operating room technician is setting up for the emergency cesarean section, while the pharmacists are coordinating the medications necessary.

Ashley Mason is the leader responsible for the quality and management of system responsiveness to urgent and emergent situations and analyzes the outcomes and functions of the teams.

The NICU team leader is the neonatal nurse practitioner who will manage the infant resuscitation. The neonatal fellow will manage the airway, the delivery neonatal nurse will dry and warm infant, and the neonatal resident will perform chest compressions if indicated. The transport nurse will place the umbilical catheters. All individual teams will have nurse recorders to document all interventions.

TABLE 9.1. Definition and Use of SBAR.

Abbreviation	Definition
S	Situation, providing the pertinent information
B	Background, issues associated with the situation
A	Assessment, clinical priorities about the situation
R	Recommendations, what's needed for successful outcomes

The coordination of the situation and clear monitoring is key to facilitate and develop a common understanding and respect of the team environment. Clearly this cannot be competitive or attitude driven. Rather, the team environment applies strategies to facilitate shared and common goals that promote successful patient outcomes and decrease patient morbidity (AHRQ 2012). In order to accomplish these goals, each team member must anticipate the needs of the other team members as if each team member were part of an orchestra and relied on each other to complete a musical symphony. This can only occur through coordinated simulated drills which Ashley facilitated on a monthly basis for smaller scale situations, and larger, system wide situations on a quarterly basis. The goal is to facilitate a well-developed respected team concept which provides a safety net for each other and the patient (JCAHO 2006). Team success is achieved through mutual support and the ability to anticipate through clinical drills, knowledge, known situations, and the ability to balance stressful pressures. The key for success includes clear, concise information and the ability to transmit information through multiple mediums that assures accuracy, reception of information, and documentation (Morey *et al.* 2002). Finally, it is important to pass on accurate information during shift relief. Use of the SBAR (Table 9.1) provides a systematic method for the continuity of patient care, maintaining patient stability, and keeping all team members informed about the patient.

Principles of Debriefing

Debriefing immediately once the patient or patients are stabilized is critical. Ashley clearly knows that all situations may not have successful outcomes. This may leave individuals with moral and ethical distress which leads to compromise in future situations and may effect not only the individual but coworkers or other patients. Being able to discuss the feelings and perceptions of team members as well as the discussion of the strengths and weaknesses of the situation is critical to the function of the team.

This required massive organization and coordination for one trauma patient that subsequently becomes two and requires inter-disciplinary coordination of not only system management but also team and individual management. In order to achieve these functional goals, there are detailed concepts that must be put into place to achieve successful outcomes, and everyone must know their role to function independently and interdependently while still functioning interdisciplinary.

Facilitating the correction of system deficiencies, workload distribution, evaluation of care, suggestions for change, or documenting situations for improvement to assure accurate recordings are critical to the successful outcomes for future patients (Pexton 2005). Not only is decreasing mortality critical, but decreasing morbidity is also critical to future patient outcomes. The debriefing should include all team members involved in the situation or discussion with each individual team. Further debriefings should include the individual team leaders to provide a forum to discuss if the process of the interdisciplinary management was facilitated. Team attitudes are critical and must be discussed and addressed respectfully of each other's autonomy and independent function. Individuals are not classified as better than others but as complementary to each other to support all the efforts of the team members (AHRQ 2008; Kotter and Rathgeber 2006).

TRANSFORMATIONAL LEADERSHIP

Transformational leaders are always visible and part of the team concept. They promote continuous commitment to the goal and demonstrate continued efforts to motivate the team. Ashley demonstrated her commitment to the vision by positive reinforcement, demonstrating rewards for successful leadership and behaviors by focusing on quality achievements, statistics, and outcome data. Transformational leaders are people oriented with and who believe in success, which comes from perseverance and deep commitment to change and improvement. This positive energy flows through passion and confidence that is supported by science, data, and the use of research methods (Bass 1990, 1985).

Transformational leaders invoke a change process which incorporate charismatic and visionary leaders to see the current process, analyze the statistics, and envision the change potential. These leaders are influential and are able to transform individuals to achieve and accomplish more than what is usually expected. The core leadership values embedded within transformational leaders include ethics, standards, emotions, and long term goals. This further encompasses understanding the needs of the individual team members, assessing and satisfying their needs, while mutually meeting the needs of the establishment. Transformational leaders can change the entire culture of the workforce through the development of a transformational process. Burns says transformational leadership, "occurs when one or more persons engage with others in such a way that leaders and followers raise one another to higher levels of motivation and morality," (1978). This leadership process views and involves individuals as personalized, distinct human beings with very specific thoughts related to motivation and morality. The leader and team members work together to raise the standard of care, increase morality, and promote ethical principles, and are engaged in team goals (Northouse 2012; Tichy and Ulrich 1984).

As a transformational leader, Ashley was focused on changing the facility's values to reflect not only moral and ethical values but to decrease patient morbidity and mortality. Transformational leaders demonstrate charisma, which is a specific quality that has captivating effects on their followers (House 1976). A charismatic leader is dominant with a desire to influence, and demonstrates confidence and strong values. A charismatic leader exhibits competence, strong role modeling, excellent communication skills with high expectations, and an expression of confidence and motivation. These characteristics and behaviors have an effect on team members to trust in the leader's ideology. Team members development a congruence of beliefs between them and the leader, become emotionally involved, and promote accountability among all team members.

These leaders demonstrate a strong set of internal values and are effective in motivating team members to enlist the greater good over self satisfaction. Transformational leaders forge the link by emphasizing intrinsic success and extrinsic factors. This facilitates the transformation of team member's self concepts and identity and expresses high expectations of the members while enlisting self confidence and self efficacy (Shamir *et al.* 1993). Transformational leaders influence others with charisma; they inspire motivation, intellectual, stimulation, and individual creativity. Other leadership styles, such as transactional leaders, invoke contingent rewards based on active or passive corrective transactions (Northouse 2012).

Concepts Related to Transformational Leadership

The principles associated with transformational leadership include the concept of "idealized influence charisma." This type of charisma uses strong role models who identify with these leaders and emulate their ethical values. Team members respect the leader and facilitate the vision and sense of mission. A second concept includes "inspirational motivation" which is defined as a way to inspire team members through motivation and commitment toward a shared vision. The transformational leader uses symbols and emotional appeal to achieve team spirit. The third concept includes "intellectual stimulation" which inspires team members through creative innovation and challenges to their own beliefs. The transformational leader supports the team members by facilitating new ideas and by developing innovative resolutions to organizational challenges. Further, the transformational leader provides "individual consideration" and supports a climate that attends to individual team member needs. Transformational leaders follow Maslow's hierarchy and encourage individuals toward self-actualization to promote a successful team. These methods do not entail a focus on individual or personal development, but rather on the concept of self development for team success or institutional success, thus facilitating increasing quality and safety (Northouse 2012).

According to Kouzes and Pozner (2002), transformational leaders model the way through exemplary leadership by establishing a personal example with their individual behaviors and by inspiring a shared vision that challenge others to transcend the "status quo." Transformational leaders challenge the process to improve, are willing to take risks, and manage change, while creating an environment that establishes a feeling of self worth and pride in the outcomes of the work environment. To achieve improvements, these leaders authenticate success through outcomes data, the establishment of benchmarks, and the encouragement and refinement of goals when failures exist. Leaders such as Ashley empower and nurture team members, stimulate change by being strong role models, commonly create a vision, and require leadership team members to build trust, foster collaboration, and futuristic visions.

SUMMARY POINTS

- Successful teams require organization and a systematic approach to communication, leadership, and patient outcomes.
- Teamwork competencies include strong leadership skills that involve the ability to direct and coordinate team members, assign roles, motivate team members, and facilitate optimal team performance.
- The coordination of a clinical situation and clear monitoring is key to facilitate and develop a common understanding and respect of the team environment.
- Transformational leaders promote continuous commitment to the goal and demonstrate continued efforts to motivate the team.

- Transformational leaders influence others with charisma, and inspire motivation, intellectual stimulation, and individual creativity.
- Transformational leaders empower and nurture team members and stimulate change by being strong role models, commonly creating a vision, and requiring leadership team members to build trust, foster collaboration, and futuristic visions.

REFERENCES

Agency for Healthcare Research and Quality (AHRQ). 2008. *The Quick Reference Guide to TeamSTEPPS® Action Planning: TeamSTEPPS® Implementation Guide.* Agency for Healthcare Research and Quality, Rockville, MD. http://www.ahrq.gov/professionals/education/curriculum-tools/TeamSTEPPS®/instructor/essentials/implguide3.html

Awad, S.S., S.P. Fagan, C. Bellows, D. Albo, *et al.* 2005. Bridging the communication gap in the operating room with medical team training. *Am J Surg 190*(5):770–4.

Baker, D.P., S. Gustafson, J. Beaubien, E. Salas, and P. Barach. 2005. Medical teamwork and patient safety: The evidence-based relation. Literature review (Contract No. 282-98-0029, Task Order #54 to the American Institutes for Research). AHRQ Publication No. 05-0053. Rockville, MD. Agency for Healthcare Research and Quality.

Bass, B.M. 1985. *Leadership and performance beyond expectation.* New York: Free Press.

Bass, B.M. 1990. From transactional to transformational leadership: Learning to share the vision. *Organizational Dynamics*, (Winter): 19–31.

Burns, J.M. 1978. *Leadership.* New York: Harper & Row.

Haig, K., S. Sutton, and J. Whittington. 2006. SBAR: A shared mental model for improving communication between clinicians. *Jt Comm J Qual Patient Saf 32*(3):167–75.

House, R.J. 1976. A 1976 Theory of Charismatic Leadership. In *Leadership: The Cutting Edge* (189–207). Hunt, J.G. and L.L. Larson, Eds.. Carbondale: Southern Illinois University Press. http://www.nwlink.com/~donclark/leader/transformational_leadership.html#sthash.VuuwuWud.dpuf

Kohn, L.T., J.M. Corrigan, and M.S. Donaldson, Eds. 2000. *To err is human: Building a safer health system.* Washington, DC: Committee on Quality of Health Care in America, Institute of Medicine, National Academy Press.

Kotter, J. and H. Rathgeber. 2006. *Our iceberg is melting: Changing and succeeding under adverse conditions.* St. Martin's Press.

Kouzes, J.M. and B.Z. Posner. 2002. *The Leadership Challenge, 3rd ed.* Jossey-Bass.

Joint Commission on Accreditation of Healthcare Organizations (JCAHO). 2006. *Patient safety: Essentials for healthcare, 4th ed.* Oakbrook Terrace, Ill: Joint Commission Resources, Inc.

Mann, S., R. Marcus, and B. Sachs. 2006. Lessons from the cockpit: How team training can reduce errors on L&D. (Grand Rounds) *Contemporary Ob/Gyn* v51 i1:34(8).

Northouse, P.G. 2012. *Leadership Theory and Practice.* Sage Publication. http://www.sagepub.com/northouse6e/main.htm

Pexton, C. 2005. *Establishing a framework for organization transformation in healthcare.* GE Healthcare Performance Solutions.

Pronovost, P., S. Berenholtz, T. Dorman, P.A. Lipsett, T. Simmonds, and C. Haraden. 2003. Improving communication in the ICU using daily goals. *J Crit Care 18*(2):71–5.

Shamir, B., R. House, and M. Arthur. 1993. *The Motivational Effects of Charismatic Leadership: A Self-Concept Based Theory Organization Science* Vol. 4, No. 4(577–594). INFORMS. http://www.jstor.org/stable/2635081

Tichy, N.M. and D.O. Ulrich. 1984. The Leadership Challenge—A Call for the Transformational Leader. In *Classical Readings of Organizational Behavior* (2008), Ott, Parkes, and Simpson, Eds. Belmont, CA: Thomson-Wadsworth.http://www.nwlink.com/~donclark/leader/transformational_leadership.html#sthash.VuuwuWud.dpuf

Defining Clinical Scholarship

DENISE M. KORNIEWICZ PHD., RN, FAAN

Chapter 10 presents the principles of clinical scholarship. An example of a complicated case study about a patient problem is presented and how to apply the principles of evidence-based practice approaches is used.

Case Presentation

J.S. has been a family nurse practitioner for over 2 years and has worked in the diabetes specialty center managing diabetic patients. Most recently, she has had an increase in the number of middle-aged women who have been noncompliant in their treatment regimens. As a result, J.S. decided to review the best clinical options available in order to improve her ability to assist similar patients in their compliance and treatment of type 2 diabetes. M.A. is one of J.S.'s typical cases that she manages.

M.A. is a 50-year-old woman with a 1-year history of type 2 diabetes. Although she was diagnosed in 2012, she had symptoms indicating hyperglycemia for 2 years prior to diagnosis. She has had fasting blood glucose records indicating values of 118–127 mg/dl, which were described to her as "borderline diabetes."

During a routine physical, M.A.'s family physician noted that she recently gained weight and had pain in her right foot. She has been on metformin, 500 mg BID, however she has not been compliant in routinely taking her medications. M.A. stated that sometimes she forgets to keep medication available especially if she goes out to eat.

M.A. does not routinely test her blood glucose levels at home and often states that she is going to lose weight to control her blood glucose. M.A. states that her elderly mother has diabetes and she does not understand why she has it since she does not overly indulge in sugar products. In fact, M.A. rarely eats candy, although she does enjoy eating cakes and some pies.

During the past year, M.A. has gained 35 lbs. even though she has remained active by exercising and routinely walking. Additionally, her current job required her to stand for long periods of time with only three short breaks during the day to rest. Most recently she noticed that her left foot would swell and a small wound appeared on her instep. She has experience pain in that area and it seems to be aggravated by her constant standing.

M.A.'s diet reveals a propensity for desserts, minimal bread, and some pasta. She has seen a dietician and is aware of how carbohydrates affect her blood sugar. She snacks intermittently but tries to eat healthy food during the week such as chicken and fish. M.A. does not smoke and drinks less than 8 oz. of wine a week.

M.A. is seeking care today because her hemoglobin A1c has never been greater than 7.2 but is now 8.0. Her blood pressure is borderline ranging between 128/70–144/90. Although she was told that her blood pressure was "a little high," she did not want to be prescribed any antihypertensive medication because she felt if she lost weight it would go back to normal.

M.A. was recently seen by her family practice doctor because of her foot pain and open wound. She was initially hospitalized for wound management and antibiotic therapy a year ago but now only experiences pain. She recovered without any issues and returned to work after being instructed in preventive foot care. M.A.'s medical records also indicate that she had one C-section and no other hospitalizations related to the foot problem. All of her immunizations are up to date, and, in general, she has been remarkably healthy for many years.

M.A. presented with uncontrolled type 2 diabetes and a complex set of comorbidities, all of which needed treatment (hypertension, obesity, peripheral vascular disease). J.S. decided that her first task was to prioritize M.A's care by selecting the most pressing healthcare issue. Although M.A. stated that she needed to lose weight, her major concern for seeking diabetes specialty care was her elevated glucose levels; her hypertension also needed to be addressed.

As an APN, J.S. is suited to work with M.A. on further educating her about the self-management of diabetes as well as assisting her with becoming more compliant with her medications. J.S. knows that M.A. will only respond to her treatment plan if she takes responsibility for her own health needs. In order to determine the best next steps in the management of M.A.'s health issues., J.S. embarks on seeking the best evidence-based practice guidelines that support her clinical decisions.

ESSENTIALS OF EVIDENCE-BASED CLINICAL PRACTICE

In an effort to provide a framework for safe, efficient, and effective clinical care, the Institute of Medicine (IOM 2003) re-evaluated patient-centered practice and adapted the use of evidence-based clinical guidelines as the scientific underpinnings for clinical care. The report from IOM (2003) suggested that healthcare professionals define evidence-based practice (EBP) and provide the best evidence for their decisions to problem-solving patient interventions. Today, the most widely and acceptable definition for EBP has been adapted from Sackett *et al.* as, "conscientious, judicious, and explicit use of current best evidence in making decisions about the care of the individual patients," (1996). The primary component to this process is to use the best scientific evidence available for individuals or populations and to make informed and safe decisions about the healthcare that is rendered.

J.S. has been a family nurse practitioner for over 2 years and has worked in the diabetes specialty center managing diabetic patients. Most recently, she has had an increase in the number of middle-aged women who have been noncompliant in their treatment regimens. As a result, J.S. decided to review the best clinical options available in order to improve her ability to assist similar patients in their compliance and treatment of type 2 diabetes.

Elements of Evidence-Based Practice

There are four essential steps that are used to evaluate or implement an evidence-based clinical practice approach: (1) development of the clinical question, (2) review of the evidence in the literature, (3) critically appraising the validity of the research completed on the topic, and (4) applying the findings to make a clinical decision. Often, clinicians have difficulty defining the specific clinical question. For example, in our case study an appropriate clinical question may be: what factors impact noncompliant, middle-aged diabetic women? Embedded within the clinical question is the population of interest, age, gender, and clinical diagnosis. Thus, once the clinical question is formulated, then it becomes easier to develop a comprehensive review of the literature that would include the best evidence available for treatment interventions.

A comprehensive review of the literature includes an understanding of the levels of evidence available for the clinical problem. One way to guide a scientific search is to categorize the scientific review into a hierarchy consisting of level I as the strongest and level VI as the weakest. The levels of evidence are important since the higher levels reflect greater scientific rigor such as systematic reviews, mega-analysis, or clinical guidelines. The lower levels consist of case reports or expert opinions and often are not as scientifically determined. The stronger the evidence leads clinicians to make safer clinical decisions that are more reliable and accurate (Facchiano and Snyder 2012).

Once a review of literature related to the clinical problem has been completed and the literature is systematically leveled, the clinician should begin the process of critical appraisal. The critical appraisal process involves the evaluation of the scientific and nonscientific research that has been conducted about the clinical problem. It is not a judgment process, rather it includes the quality of the research or data that has been provided. Also it includes what worked and what did not work based on the patients' condition.

> M.A. is a 50-year-old woman with a 1-year history of type 2 diabetes. Although she was diagnosed in 2012, she had symptoms indicating hyperglycemia for 2 years prior to diagnosis. She has had fasting blood glucose records indicating values of 118–127 mg/dl, which were described to her as "borderline diabetes."
>
> During a routine physical, M.A.'s family physician noted that she recently gained weight and had pain in her right foot. She has been on metformin, 500 mg BID, however she has not been compliant in routinely taking her medications. M.A. stated that sometimes she forgets to keep medication available especially if she goes out to eat.

The critical appraisal determines the validity of the findings based on how the results were applied. For example, in the case study, findings associated with diabetes among middle-age women and compliance to medications would be examined. The rationale for investigating this issue would be to look for sufficient details about participants who were most like the patient population represented. Validity includes how the objectives of the study were met, how clear the findings were from multiple databases, and whether or not multiple authors were able to assess the quality of the findings. If the APN is going to make a clinical decision about which intervention(s) to use, it is important to find outcomes consistent with the patient population that is being explored (Melynk and Fineout-Overholt 2011).

Finally, application of the findings includes the APN's ability to determine the best clinical interventions necessary for treating the patient. Often, clinical decisions include a problem-solving process that involves the integration of old and new knowledge. However, the ability to synthesize all the scientific evidence available for a variety of clinical problems can be complex. Nevertheless, it is the APNs critical thinking skills that provide a scientific framework to investigate each of the patient's presenting problems.

> M.A. presented with uncontrolled type 2 diabetes and a complex set of comorbidities, all of which needed treatment (hypertension, obesity, peripheral vascular disease). J.S. decided that her first task was to prioritize M.A.'s care by selecting the most pressing healthcare issue. Although M.A. stated that she needed to lose weight, her major concern for seeking diabetes specialty care was her elevated glucose levels; her hypertension also needed to be addressed.

For complex patient problems, the APN should keep four criteria in mind when reviewing the scientific evidence available. These principles include (1) soundness of the evidence-based approach, (2) comprehensiveness and specificity, (3) ease of use, and (4) availability (Guyatt *et al.* 2008). By using an EBP approach to solving patient care processes, better patient relationships and shared decision-making can occur. As a result, the more positive patient outcomes will provide the scientific platform for the future healthcare system.

CLINICAL DECISION-MAKING USING EBP

Clinical decision making has been defined as a balance of experience, knowledge, and information gathering by using assessment skills to guide a clinician's ability to make a decision based on the best available clinical practice evidence (Chapa *et al.* 2012). There are several competencies that have been used to assist clinicians with the development of an effective clinical decision. These competencies include core values and skills such as (1) pattern recognition, (2) critical thinking, (3) communication, (4) use of evidence-based approaches, (5) teamwork, (6) the ability to share results, and (7) the use of reflection (Table 10.1).

Often, APNs have to integrate these skills while problem-solving a clinical patient case, and the outcomes associated with the patient's care may vary from simple to complex.

TABLE 10.1. *Core Skills for Effective Clinical Decisions (Royal College of Nursing 2012).*

Core Skill	Definition
Pattern recognition	Learning from clinical experience
Critical thinking	Ability to examine assumptions, recognition of personal attitudes, ability to evaluate the evidence
Communication	Active listening, patient-centered approach
Evidence-based approach	Uses available evidence and clinical practice guidelines
Team work	Gathers evidence from others, advice from colleagues
Sharing	Reflects on decision to improve care
Reflection	Obtains feedback and outcomes associated with the care

J.S. knows that M.A. will only respond to her treatment plan if she takes responsibility for her own health needs. In order to determine the best next steps in the management of M.A., J.S. embarks on seeking the best evidence-based practice guidelines that support her clinical decisions.

Clinical decisions can range from fast, intuitive decisions to well thought out, reasoned, or evidence based. Often the spectrum of decision-making includes the ability to differentiate between the simple to complex while solving a clinical event. There are many factors associated with clinical decision-making and each skill has the potential to impact the effectiveness of a decision. Ideally, clinical decisions would be based on objective clinical data that has been proven to provide the best possible patient outcomes. However, the reality of clinical practice situations has demonstrated that APNs have to make a decision in a hectic clinical environment using their knowledge, skills, and experience to make the best possible decision while ensuring that the outcome is the safest for the patient. Traynor *et al.* (2012) has demonstrated that when healthcare providers are interrupted or if the environment is busy or hectic, clinical decisions can be marginalized. Nevertheless, the best clinical decisions are based on knowledge about the clinical evidence, knowing one's own competencies, and knowing the patient. APNs who base their clinical knowledge on current practice guidelines, understand their own limitations, and are familiar with the needs of the patient are considered safe, reliable, and competent practitioners.

The application of EBP undergirds the ability of the APN to integrate the clinical knowledge with the overall clinical decision to determine the best evidence-based patient outcome. APNs need to focus their attention on the critical analysis and integration of the best evidence to ensure high quality patient care. Often, the use of electronic databases has been provided in the clinical setting to assist the clinician with pre-appraised research sources to facilitate a clear decision. Depending on the resources available, the comprehensiveness of the data source, and the ability to access and make comparisons about a clinical decision determines the comprehensiveness of the clinical decision. Stubbings *et al.* (2012) found that clinical decisions were based on three major situational themes: individual factors influencing the situation, interpersonal behaviors influencing the situation, and the situation's impact on improving working relationships and patient care.

Weber (2007) reported that APN practices that used a clinical decision system accessed the database to review the forecasted patient outcomes and compared this information to their judgment. This provided a method to review consistency for potential patient decisions. Perhaps the use of a clinical systems support model would assist APNs with additional information that can be shared with the patient and family members. Use of this technology would provide a platform that integrates the knowledge and skills of the APN as well as "state of the art" data necessary for the patient and family members to be well-informed consumers or participants in their overall treatment.

DEVELOPMENT OF CLINICAL SCHOLARSHIP

The development and sophistication of future clinical scholarship will depend on the continued critical use of scientific databases that probe the clinical question and provide the best clinical solutions. Population-based healthcare will require proof of data that demonstrates that what we do affects the outcome of the patient. Therefore, the future role of the APN will be to provide the clinical knowledge necessary to improve patient outcomes.

The essentials of doctoral education (ACCE 2008) have provided the framework for educating APNs. Clinical scholarship includes the integration of facts and the synthesis of knowledge. The clinical scholar applies the knowledge to solve a problem and develops new ways to disseminate knowledge to others. APNs will lead the way to further the development of science and meet the needs of patients through the discovery of new methods for the prevention and treatment of disease. APNs will engage in advancing nursing practice by providing change and leadership for evidence-based clinical care. As APNs translate practice changes into health systems, the overall quality of patient care will improve. Thus, APNs will be recognized as the clinical change agents of the future since their scholarship will involve the integration of practice from diverse sources and across disciplines.

The ability to collaborate across and between health disciplines includes the application of new competencies which translate research into practice. The clinical scholar evaluates practice models and works within multidisciplinary settings that foster teamwork and the clinical analysis of patient outcomes. The ability to foster population-based care that implements prevention and activities to improve the health status of the population will be an essential characteristic for future APN scholars. The APN clinical scholar will make clinical practice recommendations that guide practice based on the determinants of health, environmental changes, cultural diversity, and interventions that are endorsed by representatives from multiple disciplines.

SUMMARY POINTS

- The use of EBP will require the best scientific evidence available to produce the best patient outcomes and quality care.
- The quality of EBP includes expert scientific data related to a clinical problem.
- Clinical decision-making includes competencies that promote expert problem solving skills.
- The science of clinical decision-making requires the scientific knowledge necessary for the development of clinical practice guidelines.
- Clinical scholarship includes the application of EBP methods that impact on the quality of population-based healthcare.

REFERENCES

APRN Report. Consensus Model for APRN: Licensure, Accreditation, Certification and Education. Accessed July 7, 2008. www.aacn.nche.edu/education resources/ APRN Report.pdf

Chapa, D., M. Hartung, L. Mayberry, and C. Pintz. 2013. Using preappraised evidence sources to guide practice decisions. *Journal of the American Association of Nurse Practitioners 25* (234–243).

Facchiano, L. and C. Snyder. 2012. Evidence-based practice for the busy nurse practitioner: Part two: Searching for the best evidence to clinical inquiries. *Journal of the American Academy of Nurse Practitioners, 24* (640–648).

Guyatt, Drummond, M.O. Mead, and D. Cook. 2008. *User's guide to the medical literature: A manual for evidence-based clinical practice 2nd ed.* New York, NY; Mc-Graw Hill.

Melynk and E. Fineout-Overholt. 2011. *Evidence-based practice in nursing and healthcare, a guide to best practice* (2nd ed.). Philadelphia, PA; Lippincott Williams & Wilkins.

Patient Safety: Achieving a New Standard of Care. 2003. Institute of Medicine. National Academy of Science, Washington, DC.

Royal College of Nursing. 2012. *Advanced Nurse Practitioners: An RCN Guide to Advanced Nursing Practice*, Advanced Nurse Practitioners and Programme Accreditation. RCN, London.

Sackett, D., W. Rosenberg, J. Gray, R. Haynes, and W. Richardson. 1996. Evidence-based medicine: What it is and what it isn't: It's about integrating individual clinical expertise and the best external evidence. *British Medical Journal, 3*(12) (71–72).

Stubbings, L., W. Chaboyer and A. McMurray. 2012. Nurses' use of situation awareness in decision-making: an integrative review. *Journal of Advanced Nursing 68* (7) (1443–1453).

Traynor M., M. Boland, and N. Buus. 2010. Autonomy, evidence and intuition: nurses and decision-making. *Journal of Advanced Nursing 66*(7) (1584–1591).

Becoming an Expert Clinical Scholar

DENISE M. KORNIEWICZ PHD., RN, FAAN

The Chapter 11 case study emphasizes the expertise needed to be an advance practice clinical scholar. Topics include dissemination of clinical scholarship, peer review, publication, mentorship, and recognition of clinical expertise.

Case Presentation

Dawn always wanted to be a nurse. In fact, Dawn would "play" nurse at an early age and she was excited to get admitted to a 4 year nursing program after graduating from high school. Dawn successfully completed her baccalaureate program in nursing and passed her state boards. Once she was fully licensed she was mentored as a staff nurse in the emergency room of a major medical hospital. Dawn loved learning from her fellow staff nurse mentors and cherished her clinical work. However, within 3 years, she yearned to learn more. While working as a nurse manager, she decided that she enjoyed teaching patients, mentoring new graduates, and being part of a clinical decision team. Often, she felt that she needed to learn more about team leadership and decided to pursue a graduate degree.

During her formal graduate nursing education, Dawn became an adult nurse practitioner and learned that clinical decision-making outcomes forced her to become more of an expert since she was now responsible for handing a case load of patients and assisting them to take control of their own health and assist in their own health management. Dawn worked for the next 5 years as an adult nurse practitioner along side a family practice physician, a physician assistant, and an internal medicine physician. She learned that her colleagues respected her because she took the time to become an expert in the management of adult health problems. Because her caseload included a variety of acute and chronic health conditions, Dawn learned to seek additional knowledge from her peers as well as to attend regional and national conferences so that she could build her clinical knowledge base. Often the programs she attended were multidisciplinary so she learned to work well with her peers and respect their knowledge as they respected hers.

Dawn was well respected by her physician colleagues as well as by other nurse practitioners that had similar clinical practice experience. Because of her increased clinical skills she was asked to teach other beginning nurse practitioners as well medical school students. During the next few years in her career, Dawn was quite content because she was becoming an expert at managing patients with chronic disease such as hypertension, diabetes, and seasonal health problems. Dawn had been practicing well over 5 years as an adult nurse practitioner, teaching both medical students, nurse practitioners, and physician assistant students. With the changes occurring in healthcare reimbursement and the consolidation of healthcare systems, Dawn's initial primary care practice had been purchased into a group primary care practice. Now she was as part of the local medical hospital and she was asked to work with more healthcare professionals from other disciplines and to teach a variety of students providing primary care services and assisting with the development of standardized clinical protocols.

It was during Dawn's 12th year as a nurse practitioner that she began to see more complicated patients and was asked to take on increased responsibilities with the primary care practice. For example, she was asked to cover in the primary care outreach clinic, to make primary care rounds at the local rehabilitation center, and to cover a geriatric clinic on Saturday mornings. As a result of her increased practice responsibilities and her thirst to improve her own knowledge, she returned to graduate school to earn her doctorate of nursing practice (DNP) degree. While enrolled in the program, Dawn was challenged to complete quality assurance projects, to develop clinical protocols based on evidence-based practice trends, and to develop papers associated with healthcare policy. Within 2 years, Dawn graduated from the program with new knowledge and advanced expertise in the management of adult health patients. Soon not only her colleagues, but also her patients and others were viewing Dawn as an expert mentor and expert clinician outside of the immediate community.

As Dawn continued to practice as a nurse practitioner and expert clinical teacher she was asked to participate as a contributing author on several clinical papers. Initially, Dawn did not see herself as a writer, nor did she view herself as anyone who was any different from her peers. Due to her work with her colleagues, she found that she was able to write about patients that she managed as well as suggest new treatment regimens all within the scope of clinical practice. In fact, her original work was beginning to be used by other nurse practitioners and she found that she was quoted or cited by others for her clinical outcome protocols. Dawn was happy with her accomplishments and was helpful to new nurse practitioner students who were hesitant to make decisions or to publish. Often, Dawn would be called upon to render an opinion about a new treatment mode or was asked to implement a clinical practice change based on data she would gather from her patients. Dawn was becoming a clinical scholar since she was developing new ideas, using evidence-based research to make clinical decisions, and publishing clinical practice outcomes that impacted improving patient care. Additionally, Dawn was working in a collaborative environment that helped her pursue new clinical treatment methods. As a result, Dawn was demonstrating that clinical scholarship not only has value but also provides the foundation to improve patient care outcomes.

ESSENTIAL CONTENT FOR DEFINING CLINICAL SCHOLARSHIP

Clinical scholarship for the discipline of nursing has been defined in a variety of ways. Historically, scholarship in clinical nursing practice was defined as the processes in which patients were cared for. Nursing practice was based on the essentials of the nursing process that included the components of assessment, diagnosis, planning, implementation, and evaluation. Traditionally, nurses were concerned about process standards and guidelines versus outcomes associated with effective therapeutics. However, as the practice of nursing developed and nurse practitioners evolved, the science of clinical decision making as well as the evaluation of patient outcomes became evident when providing care for patients. No longer were nursing interventions based on whether or not the process of care was appropriate, rather, interventions were based on the scientific evidence associated with the treatment options available for patients. Thus, the understanding of clinical scholarship began to take form from simple to complex interventions to the evaluation of the science associated with evidence-based therapeutic interventions and their relationship to the patient's outcome.

> While working as a nurse manager, she decided that she enjoyed teaching patients, mentoring new graduates, and being part of a clinical decision team. Often, she felt that she needed to learn more about team leadership and decided to pursue a graduate degree.

Today, clinical scholarship has been defined by the American Association of the Colleges of Nursing (AACN) (1999) as having four dimensions: discovery, teaching, application, and integration. These concepts were derived from the seminal work of Ernest Boyer (1990) who re-evaluated "scholarship" within the discipline of education. Boyer's work tried to expand the traditional method for evaluating faculty based on the tenants of publish or perish which was associated with the tenure processes used in academic settings. The application of Boyer's model of scholarship helps to quantify the attributes of clinical inquiry and provides a conceptual framework to define how advanced practice nurses can measure their contributions to promote evidence-based clinical care.

Clinical scholarship for advanced practice nurses as defined by AACN adapts Boyer's model to include measurable outcomes that have been suggested within each of the four domains of scholarship: discovery, teaching, application, and integration (Table 11.1).

Advance practice nurses utilize scientific evidence to improve clinical interventions and to determine the best practices for standardized clinical care. Clinical scholars are defined as advance practice nurses who systematically make observations about patient care and provide the evidence needed to make clinical decisions that are based on "best practice guidelines" that promote quality patient care.

> During her formal graduate nursing education, Dawn became an adult nurse practitioner and learned that clinical decision-making outcomes forced her to become more of an expert since she was now responsible for handing a case load of patients and assisting them to take control of their own health and assist in their own health management.

In order to apply the attributes of clinical scholarship, it is important to understand the role of an advance practice nurse by incorporating the scholarship of discovery, teaching, application, and integration into dai-

TABLE 11.1. Dimensions of Clinical Scholarship for Advance Practice Nurses.

Dimension of Scholarship	Definition as Defined by the American Association of Colleges of Nursing(1999)	Examples of Scholarship Dimension from Clinical Practice Settings	Measurable Outcomes Based on Clinical Expertise
Discovery	The scholarship of discovery is the inquiry that produces the disciplinary and professional knowledge that is at the very heart of academic pursuits.	• Review of literature & dissemination of literature to peers. • Presentation at grand rounds, multidisciplinary teams. • Development of new guidelines consistent with clinical specialty & patient population.	• Publication of clinical practice guideline(s). • Presentation at clinical research conferences. • Grant writing for clinical projects. • Recognized by other peers (cited in literature, keynote speaking engagements).
Teaching	Produces knowledge to support the transfer of the science and art of nursing from the expert to the novice, building bridges between the teacher's understanding and the student's learning.	• Evaluates content for curriculum for advance practice nurses. • Develops evaluation processes consistent with clinical expertise for student clinical preceptorships.	• Assists in accreditation of clinical practice programs (DNP). • Publication of evaluation processes for clinical practice.
Application	Practice is conducted through the application of nursing and related knowledge to the assessment and validation of patient care outcomes, the measurement of quality of life indicators, the development and refinement of practice protocols/strategies, the evaluation of systems of care, and the analysis of innovative health care delivery models.	• Participates in evaluation processes within healthcare system (administrative quality assurance programs, review of clinical protocols for better patient care). • Works with other healthcare providers to discuss treatment methods and "best practices."	• National certification in clinical specialty. • Peer review of products developed such as clinical protocols, guidelines, clinical pathways.
Integration	Writings and other products that use concepts and original works from nursing and other disciplines in creating new patterns, placing knowledge in a larger context, or illuminating the data in a more meaningful way.	• Develops practice guidelines consistent with specialty area. • Works with a variety of healthcare providers to provide consistent clinical care. • Reviews & updates practice protocols.	• Publication of clinical books in specialty. • Development of new healthcare delivery models. • Presentation at interdisciplinary conferences.

ly clinical practice (Table 11.1). The art of clinical scholarship includes problem solving, innovation, and creativity. The results of clinical scholarship include better patient outcomes through the dissemination of practice innovations. Inherent in the science of clinical scholarship is the value of interdisciplinary patient care and collaborative healthcare delivery models that improve patient care and further advance the discipline of advance practice nursing.

PRINCIPLES OF CLINICAL SCHOLARSHIP

The principles of clinical scholarship outline the characteristics that determine the difference between advance practice professionals who work at a "job" versus a "profession." For example, nurse practitioners who provide care to patients within their specialty, do not actively participate in the advancement of the role of the nurse practitioner, and view their work as punching a time card are not considered clinical scholars. Whereas, nurse practitioners who are actively involved in activities such as publication, presentation of clinical data, evaluation methods, development of clinical guidelines, promotion of new practice models, or the dissemination of new clinical management protocols are considered clinical scholars as defined by AACN. What is important to distinguish is the ability for advance practice nurses to be life-long learners and innovative clinical leaders. Without the generation of new knowledge, publication, or presentation of clinical changes, the advancement of the role of the nurse practitioner becomes limited. Therefore, there are several attributes that distinguish the role of the clinical scholar for advance practice. Concepts such as peer review, publication, mentorship, and recognition of one's contributions to the role of the advance practice professional will be explored.

Peer Review

The model for peer review for advance practice nurses can be defined as the critical assessment by which an individual of the same profession, experience, and work within a similar organization critically assesses their colleagues' performance in order to strengthen the quality of patient care, and to identify areas for development or improvement. Peer review can be completed in several ways such as case discussions, review of clinical management protocols, oral or written communication about new processes, or the critique of a written manuscript. Usually, peer review involves an assessment or judgment associated with the quality of care rendered and enhances the clinical expertise required to independently practice (McKay *et al.* 2007).

Because her caseload included a variety of acute and chronic health conditions, Dawn learned to seek additional knowledge from her peers as well as to attend regional and national conferences so that she could build her clinical knowledge base. Often the programs she attended were multidisciplinary so she learned to work well with her peers and respect their knowledge as they respected hers.

Peer review assists in the self-examination by the practitioner to achieve and deliver optimal quality patient care. Formal peer review processes include a designated method for assessing clinical performance such as chart audits, communication, consultation, interprofessional collaboration, teamwork, and relationship building (Briggs *et al.* 2005). Other types of peer review processes may consist of a scientific review or the oversight of a recently developed clinical protocol or manuscript. In healthcare, peer review has been shown to be an effective way to improve professional practice models, increase clinical knowledge, and facilitate changes that improve the overall quality of patient care (Doerksen 2010). Additionally, an effective peer review model can provide advance practice professionals with (1) an understanding of clinical performance as it relates to the greater organization, (2) a method to compare clinical competencies, (3) assistance in identifying healthcare professionals experiencing difficulties, and (4) aid in improving practice behaviors consistent with standardized clinical guidelines.

Dawn was well respected by her physician colleagues as well as by other nurse practitioners that had similar clinical practice experience. Because of her increased clinical skills she was asked to teach other beginning nurse practitioners as well medical school students.

It is important to note that a valid and reliable method for a peer review process promotes a culture of safety within the clinical environment. Unfortunately, a poorly designed peer review process may create a false sense of confidence when clinical data is misconstrued or interpreted as adequate when it is not, and may cause harm to patients. The accuracy of collecting clinical data that reflects evidence-based outcomes promotes safer clinical care and provides constructive feedback for advanced practice professionals. Finally, using a set of general principles to design an effective peer review process (Table 11.2) may assist advance practice nurses to strive to continuously improve the overall quality of patient care.

TABLE 11.2. *List of Principles for a Peer Review Process.*

1. Administrators of healthcare organization support a peer review process.
2. Clinical practitioners actively engage in a peer review process as part of their practice.
3. Data processes for peer review are accurate, valid, and reliable.
4. Peer reviews are fair, equitable, legal, and ethical.
5. The outcomes from peer review processes should improve patient care.
6. Peer review processes are timely, scheduled, and include all healthcare professionals.
7. Constructive feedback is provided to participating healthcare professionals.
8. Clinical practice changes are made based on the data derived from the review of clinical decisions within the practice.
9. An annual review of a provider's clinical credentials that demonstrate improvement or changes in the provider's scope of practice is conducted.
10. An annual review of accountability measures for safe clinical practice within the organization is conducted.

Due to her work with her colleagues, she found that she was able to write about patients that she managed as well as suggest new treatment regimens all within the scope of clinical practice. In fact, her original work was beginning to be used by other nurse practitioners and she found that she was quoted or cited by others for her clinical outcome protocols.

Publication

Advance practice professionals continue to influence the quality of patient care. It is through the publication of content associated with evidence-based research beyond its original work that the transfer of clinical knowledge occurs (Harrington 2011). For example, when others cite or reference an original clinical data-based manuscript and apply it to a clinically relevant journal, the findings are more readily disseminated into clinical practice. Thus, for research-based articles, advance practice professionals need to understand the importance of publication and the utilization of research findings. Often, clinically competent advance practice nurses are hesitant to publish since they do not view themselves as clinical scholars or feel worthy of their ability to contribute to the science of clinical practice. However, in order for advance practice nurses to be recognized as peers among other health professionals, it is important to incorporate the principles of scientific publication within a professional practice model.

Dawn was happy with her accomplishments and was helpful to

new nurse practitioner students who were hesitant to make decisions or publish.

The preparation of a clinically focused, scientific manuscript requires adherence to a set of general guidelines for successful publication. These guidelines should include: authorship, acknowledgements, content, abstract, and references (Table 11.3). Once the manuscript is logically outlined, it is best to determine an appropriate journal for submission of the manuscript for publication. A few important points to consider when selecting a journal would be (1) peer review processes, (2) readership (academic, clinical, interdisciplinary), (3) impact factor (reputation, timeliness), and (4) frequency of publication (monthly, bimonthly, weekly, online availability). Last, adapting a title that clearly summarizes the intent of your publication is important. Hays (2010) suggests that keeping the title simple and informative yet stylish may be a few principles to guide an author. Perhaps focusing the title as a scientific versus a clinical paper will assist in determining the readership and provide clarity for the title. Each word in the title should focus on the content of the manuscript as well as its overall intent. Since the title is used for literature searches, cataloging, or citations, it is important to choose a title that is direct, to the point, and that reflects the most significant content that demonstrates the importance of the manuscript's content.

Often, Dawn would be called upon to render an opinion about a new treatment mode or asked to implement a clinical practice change based on data she would gather from her patients.

Mentorship

The term mentor has been defined as a guardian, advisor, or teacher (Harrington 2011). Since the inception of the advance practice role, nurse practitioners have been serving as mentors to other healthcare professionals as clinical preceptors and clinical experts providing clinical guest lectures or seminars. Often, the definition or expectation about what a mentor does, who they are, or how a person evolves as an expert mentor are issues that are not formally taught during one's formal educational program. Rather, like most practiced disciplines, the attributes of a mentor are learned on the job or by trial and error. For the discipline of advanced practice nursing, mentorship requires both formal and informal learning methods that provide a framework to understand the complexities of a mentor-mentee relationship. These components include characteristics of a good mentor,

TABLE 11.3. *Guidelines for Writing a Publishable Manuscript.*

Guideline	Definition	Example
Authorship	*First author*: responsible for idea, develops outline of paper, determines coauthors	Principal investigator on study / Initiates idea or clinical expert
	Second author: contributes to content or specialty area, writes portion of paper	Statistician, assisted in analysis of paper or specialist & contributed expertise
	Third/last author: contributes to written areas or paper, may be mentor or more senior author, final edits of paper	Professor who assisted in editing paper / Mentor or colleague
Acknowledgements	*Funding agency*: government or private agency that sponsored research, foundation, corporation	National Institutes of Health; Centers for Disease Control & Prevention; Kellogg Foundation; Johnson & Johnson
	May include primary individuals involved in the collection data or review of paper	Research assistants or students involved in the basic science research course (list names)
Content	*Scientific structure*: review of literature, methods, results, discussion	Title reflect scientific emphasis such as "A randomized study to determine pain management options" (Nursing Research, Journal of Clinical Research)
	Clinical structure: description of reports, general treatment methods, pros and cons of treatment	*Clinical title*: "Determination of treatment options for pain control based on best practice methods" (Journal of Nursing Education and Practice, American Journal of Nursing)
Abstract	*Scientific paper*: reflects subheadings in a systematic manner such as background, methods, results, and discussion	Scientific Journals such as New England Journal of Medicine, Lancet
	Clinical paper: narrative with subheadings associated with overall content of paper such as case report and discussion of best practices	*Clinical Journals such as*: Nursing Clinics of North America, Clinical Scholarship
References	Cited specifically from original or secondary sources with author, title, year, journal, volume, & page numbers	Korniewicz, D. and M. El-Masri. 2012. Exploring the benefits of double gloving during surgery. *AORN* 95(3) (328–335).
	Online references must be cited as to date retrieved as well as website used	American Association of Colleges of Nursing. Position Statement. 1999. Retrieved November 20, 2013. http://www.aacn.nche.edu/publications/position/defining-scholarship

phases of the mentor-mentee relationship, and continued role development of the expert mentor.

Several general themes associated with the characteristics of a good mentor across healthcare disciplines have been noted throughout the literature (AANP 2006; Wilson *et al.* 2013). These attributes include: facilitating goals, active listening, understanding, prioritizing practice issues, goal setting, demonstrating role modeling behaviors (communication, confidence, and values), clinical knowledge, and the recognition of one's own limitations. What is interesting to note is that most advanced practice professionals were able to identify these characteristics during their own clinical preceptorships while enrolled in their program of study. However, once in the workforce, both nurse practitioners and physician assistants lacked mentorship at their home institution (Oermann *et al.* 2010). Areas of mentorship that were missing included (1) support from other advance practice professionals, (2) office politics, (3) organizational infrastructure, (4) contract negotiations, and (5) professional relationships. Perhaps once advance practice professionals enter into the workplace, a clinical colleague should be designated as a professional practice mentor to provide further transition and role development for the advance practice practitioner.

The development of the mentor-mentee relationship may be summarized into four phases: (1) initiation of the relationship, (2) working and collaboration, (3) termination or independence, and (4) professional acceptance/mutual respect (Table 11.4). During each of these phases, both the mentor and the mentee achieve specific goals, determine mutual respect for each other, and establish a collaborative relationship that ultimately provides quality patient care. It is this synergistic working relationship that ultimately provides a model for safe clinical practice and furthers the development of clinical scholars.

Recognition of a Clinical Scholar

Advanced practice nurses' peers and other healthcare professionals are recognizing the epitome of clinical scholarship as an expert clinical scholar. For advance practice professionals, an expert clinical scholar may be defined as one who has evolved from a novice or beginner to one who has comprehensive knowledge, skills, and expertise in an area of advanced practice or clinical scholarship. Pat Benner's (1984) conceptual model describes the attributes of novice to expert for clinical nurses and can be applied to the qualities that describe advance practice practitioners. Table 11.5 defines Benner's stages of development from novice to expert as applied to the advance practice practitioner. As an advance practice nurse moves from one stage to another, the expected outcomes for clini-

TABLE 11.4. Phases of the Mentor-Mentee Relationship.

Relationship Phase	Mentor Characteristics	Mentee Characteristics
Initiation	• Establish clinical relationship, boundaries, work ethics • Develops communication style & processes	• Establish clinical relationship
Working relationships/ collaboration	• Knows strengths and weaknesses of mentee • Sets an example of professional behavior • Decreases supervision & increases management of more complicated patients	• Expresses knowledge of clinical strengths and weaknesses • Seeks collaboration when in doubt or discusses clinical practice issues about patient management • Seeks minimal professional guidance, knows when to seek help, understands one's own limitations
Termination/ independence	• Facilitates opportunities for future employment or growth	• Able to practice with minimal oversight • Completes clinical rotation competently
Professional acceptance/ mutual respect	• Provides opportunities for independence • Establishes collegial relationship by referring patients or other professionals to clinical practice	• Continues to maintain collaboration with mentor • Mutually respects clinical practice & discusses complicated patients or refers patients to mentor • Seeks advice about professional growth when needed

cal recognition become more refined and more difficult. For example, expectations associated with peer review, publication, or the generation of new clinical knowledge is considered measurable outcomes for a clinical scholar. When clinical scholars become recognized by peers within and outside of their discipline, then they have become expert clinical scholars. Often these individuals are world renown for their accomplishments and they have contributed to practice changes that have impacted a treatment method for a patient population or they have suggested prevention options that have impacted a person's life.

Dawn was becoming a clinical scholar since she was developing new ideas, using evidence-based research to make clinical decisions, and publishing clinical practice outcomes that impacted improving patient care.

TABLE 11.5. Application of Pat Benner's Model for Advance Practice Practitioners (1984).

Stages of Development	Definition	Examples of an Advance Practice Nurse's Stage of Development	Expected Outcomes Based Stage & Clinical Expertise
Novice	The novice or beginner has no experience that they are expected to perform. Lacks confidence and practice is more prolonged because of learning new role.	• New graduate from an advanced practice program. • Takes more time in the assessment of the patient.	• Reads literature consistent with safe clinical practice.
Advanced beginner	Demonstrates marginally acceptable performance because of prior clinical preceptorship during the clinical program. May have delayed time periods while providing care.	• Demonstrates acceptable beginning level skills associated with the assessment and management of patients. • Level of management is beginning to develop.	• Involved in peer review of clinical patient load. • Discusses alternate treatment methods.
Competent	Demonstrates efficiency, coordination of caseload, and has confidence in actions. Establishes a skill level consistent with the efficiency of an advance practice nurse who has been practicing 2–3 years. Patients are seen in an efficient and suitable time frame.	• Demonstrates confidence and safety by knowing when to discuss a patient's clinical problem with peers. • Carries an appropriate number of clinic patients and provides timely & proficient care.	• Provides leadership to others through clinical rounds & participates in interdisciplinary peer review. • Participates in developing clinical scholarship through development of clinical protocols or case reports.
Proficiency	Demonstrates an understanding of patient problems as a whole versus segments. The proficient advance practice practitioner learns from experience, readily suggests practice changes or interventions, and makes clear decisions based on the standards related to safe clinical practice.	• Develops new practice guidelines consistent with specialty area. • Provides leadership to other healthcare providers in the management of patient care.	• Participates in the publication of clinical manuscripts relevant to their specialty. • Leads others in the development of new healthcare delivery models. • Presentation at interdisciplinary conferences.
Expert	Demonstrates accuracy in the assessment of patient problems and is skillful at diagnosis and management. Highly skilled analytic ability is demonstrated and proficient, timely performance is demonstrated via peer review.	• Accurate diagnosis, treatment, & management of patients. • Works independently and consults only when necessary. • Teaches or precepts others.	• Particpates in all peer review processes. • Independently publishes or suggest revision of clinical protocols.

Historically, pioneers in advance practice have included such clinical scholars as Loretta Ford (2010) who started the nurse practitioner movement for independent clinical practice. Ford's initial work as a public health nurse and then as an advanced practice nurse practitioner helped define the role of the nurse practitioner in rural areas. A second example of a clinical scholar is Ruth Lubic (2013) who continues to practice as a nurse midwife in Washington, DC. Lubic is a social activist for pregnant women and developed a clinic in Washington, DC. known as the DC Developing Families Center. Her clinic provides women's health services, promotes healthy families, and demonstrates the need for continued prevention services for pregnant women. Finally, Donna Diers (1985) was a clinical scholar who advocated for the expanded scope of practice for nurse practitioners and nurse midwives. Diers' publications served as a foundation for legislation associated with the independent roles and functions of nurse practitioners.

Becoming an expert clinical scholar is a professional journey that requires constant vigilance, participation in peer review processes, and reflection on one's professional contributions toward the science of advance practice. The leadership principles necessary to be a successful expert clinical scholar include critical thinking, independence, confidence, risk taking, and the ability to be inquisitive. The expert clinical scholar is a life-long learner, engages in interdisciplinary discussions, leads others to achieve their goals, and engages novice learners into advance practice clinical models. Current and future roles that the expert clinical scholar may fulfill may include preceptor, teacher, author, primary care manager, associate within a private practice model, owner of a primary care practice, or independent primary care provider.

SUMMARY POINTS

- The principles of advance practice is based on scientific evidence associated with "best practice" guidelines.
- Clinical scholarship includes discovery, teaching, application, and integration.
- A clinical scholar understands peer review processes, participates in publications, and develops new clinical knowledge.
- Mentorship includes the ability to work with the other healthcare professionals, values collaboration, and promotes further role development.
- Expert clinical scholars are life-long learners, engaged in the discipline, and contribute to the science of advance practice.

REFERENCES

American Association of Colleges of Nursing. 1999. *Position Statement on Defining scholarship for the Discipline of Nursing.* Retrieved November 20, 2013. http://www.aacn.nche.edu/publications/position/defining-scholarship

American Academy of Nurse Practitioners (AANP). 2006. Mentoring Assessment: *Fellows of the American Academy of Nurse Practitioners Invitational Think Tank.* Retrieved November 21, 2013. http://www.aanp.org/images/documents/fellows/NPResearchRoundtable

Benner, P. 1984. *From novice to expert: Excellence and power in clinical nursing practice.* Menlo Park: Addison-Wesley (13–34).

Boyer, E.L. 1990. *Scholarship Reconsidered: Priorities of the Professoriate.* Princeton, NJ: Carnegie Foundation for the Advancement of Teaching.

Briggs, L., J. Heath, and J. Kelly. 2005. Peer review for advanced practice nurses what does it really mean? *AACN Clin, Issues 16* (1), (3–15).

Diers, D. 1985. Some conceptual and methodological issues in nurse practitioner research. *J Prof Nurs, 1* (1) (41–7).

Doerksen, K. 2010. Development and mentorship of advanced practice nurses? *Journal Prof Nurs, 26*, (3) (141–151).

Dr. Ruth Lubic Discusses Midwifery's Contribution to Improving Healthy Births. March 5, 2013. *The healthcare policy podcast.* Retrieved December 1, 2013. http://www.thehealthcarepolicypodcast.com/2013/03/listen-now.html

Ford, L. 2010. Opinions, ideas, and convictions from NPs' founding mother. *Nurse practitioner world news. 15* (11–12) (9).

Harrington, S. 2011. Mentoring new nurse practitioners to accelerate their development as primary care providers: A literature review. *Journal of the American Academy of Nurse Practitioners 23* (168–174).

Hays, J. 2010. Eight recommendations for writing titles of scientific Manuscripts, *Public Health Nursing. 27* (2) (101–103).

McKay, J., *et al.* 2007. Development and testing of an assessment instrument for the formative peer review of significant event analyses. *Quality and Safety in Health Care, 16* (2) (150–3).

Oermann, M., J. Shaw-Kokot, G. Knalfl, et al. 2010. Dissemination of research into clinical nursing literature. *Journal of Clinical Nursing, 19* (3435–3442).

Wilson, L, G. Wainwright, C. Stehly, J. Stoltzfus, and W. Hoff. 2013. Assessing the Academic and Professional Needs of Trauma Nurse Practitioners and Physician Assistants. *Journal of Trauma Nursing, 20* (1).

Transforming Clinical Practice

CAROLYN M. RUTLEDGE PHD., FNP-BC
TINA HANEY DNP, CNS
CHRISTIANNA FOWLER DNP

Chapter 12 begins with the use of current and future technology that has an impact on tracking and improving the clinical practice. A continuing case study depicts the use of technological advances that assist the APN to improve patient care in rural settings.

Case Presentation

Sally and her mother are once again in Beth's office, where Beth provides care as a family nurse practitioner. Sally is whispering that she does not know what to do. She feels alone and "over her head" in trying to care for her mother who has early stage Alzheimer's disease. Tears fall down her cheek as she expresses how she is unable to sleep at night due to her mother's wandering. As Sally tries to talk to Beth, her mother says, "That is not true. I sleep all night." Sally sighs, "I can't keep on going like this. I am exhausted and feel like I am constantly at battle with my mother. I just don't feel like anyone understands what I am going through."

After Sally and her mother leave, Beth sits in her office wondering what she can do. She can feel the pain that Sally is experiencing and notes that this type of situation keeps repeating itself. She thinks, "There has to be another way. No wonder our healthcare system is in crisis. It seems like the only solution is to try to get Sally's mother into a facility, but is that what is best for any of them?"

Beth is part of a group that is meeting to provide interprofessional healthcare education in a local university. The group consists of Beth, an ANP, a CNS, a Clinical Counselor (CC), and a Physical Therapist (PT). Beth tells her story of the "Sallies" that she has encountered. It is not surprising that many of the other group members have had similar frustrations. Specifically, the ANP had just completed her DNP Capstone Project in which she addressed the stress of "homebound caregivers." Many of the caregivers found it difficult to leave home with their elderly family member. Trips out of the house often resulted in the care recipient becoming confused and at times belligerent. It was not uncommon for the elderly individual to become lost to healthcare. Based on this experience, the GNP decided that her mission was to provide home health services. Realizing that home visits can be quite costly and time-consuming, she began seeking ways to enhance the home visit with telehealth. She saw telehealth as a mechanism for delivering care to the caregiver and the elderly family member in the privacy of their home. This would provide access in a more efficient, less frustrating, and cost-effective manner. Based on the input form Beth and the ANP, the interprofessional group decided to try to develop a new model for providing assistance to caregivers like Sally. They all agreed that this new model would be based on the utilization of technology such as telehealth.

ESSENTIAL PRINCIPLES OF TELEHEALTH

Telehealth, as defined by the U.S. Health and Human Services Administration (2012), is the use of technologies for telecommunication and the provision of electronic information for the purpose of distributing healthcare information, patient data, and healthcare services among patients and healthcare professionals. Telehealth may be used to connect the patient with healthcare professionals as well as to connect health professionals with each other. Technologies include real time videoconferencing, remote transfer of patient diagnostic and physiologic data (imaging or remote monitoring), and cell phones and mobile apps (Figure 12.1). Telehealth can be used by healthcare professionals to provide care and support through remote access to communities and populations with limited access to healthcare (Phillips 2010; U.S. Department of Health and Human Services 2008).

Telehealth consists of the use of technology to provide interprofessional collaboration, social and provider support, patient and provider education, and telemedicine (medical consultation, home healthcare monitoring, digital imaging, and videoconferencing, see Figure 12.1). Telemedicine, a subset of telehealth, encompasses primarily remote patient care (U.S. Department of Health and Human Services 2012). Information obtained from the electronic health records can be applied

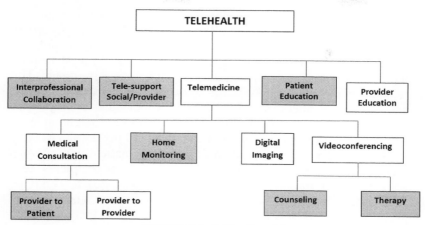

FIGURE 12.1. Telehealth model.

to telehealth. As a result, this model can be used to address the needs of the caregiver, especially when they are tasked with caring for family member.

TELESUPPORT

The CNS in the interprofessional group used telehealth to improve the care provided to caregivers of medically fragile and technology-dependent children. She had identified a disconnection between the healthcare providers, parents, and their children. Parents expressed that they felt removed and isolated from providers even though they were assigned a home health nurse. The CNS established an e-mail communication program with the parents so that they would have two-way communication. The program was structured so that weekly information relevant to caring for a medically fragile child at home was sent to parents via e-mail. Parents were encouraged to asynchronously communicate with the CNS. Examples of e-mails included concerns regarding the homecare nurse, minor issues regarding their child's care, questions about community services, and general "rants" as some parents called them. Outcomes from this program included the general parent's perceived well-being and demonstrated improved satisfaction with their care. Parent's overwhelmingly reported a sense of connection and a desire for the service to continue. Comments included "this made a difference," "continue sending e-mails," and "it's all about caring that makes a person feel better," (Haney and Adams-Tufts 2012).

While communicating with parents of homebound and medically fragile children, the CNS identified a lack of support for the siblings.

As a result of this need, she developed a closed-group Facebook page for these siblings. This was a safe place for the children to share experiences and ask questions of health professionals. While the site did have oversight by a facilitator from the home health agency, the Facebook group page was for the preteen and teenage siblings, not parents. This provided a safe place for the siblings to connect and share their stories and thoughts with other teens that could really understand the joys, frustrations, and fears of having a sibling that requires constant home care.

Studies have shown that the Internet and social media such as blogging, Twitter, and Facebook, when designed for patient and provider support, enhances social connection and improves the recipients' feelings of support (Clifton *et al.* 2013; McDaniel *et al.* 2012). The types of interventions provided by the CNS using e-mail and Facebook communication with a patient and/or caregiver is unique in that the participants can receive support in the comfort of their homes from reputable healthcare professionals. This is especially vital in that much of the information available to patients and their caregivers on the Internet can be misleading. It is imperative that providers take the lead in establishing reputable sites that provide accurate and beneficial information. Providers must also stay current with the changing trends and popularity of various social media platforms. For example, in 2013 there were 1.15 billion Facebook users, 500 million twitter users, 500 million plus who signed onto Google daily, 1 billion YouTube visitors, and 46% of web users turn to social media for advice (Social Media Today 2013). Recent studies have shown that 4.2 million people use a mobile device to access social media sites (Social Media Today 2013) thereby allowing them quick connection and access from any location.

TELE-EDUCATION

During the interprofessional group meeting, Beth discussed the need to provide education to patients in rural settings. She felt frustrated that there was a void in the education as identified in a study she conducted with one of her students whose specialty area was stroke management. The student worked in a university's stroke center that was using telemedicine to provide stroke consultation to emergency departments (EDs) as far as 300 miles away. When a patient came to the rural hospital with stroke symptoms, the ED staff would transmit the patient's images to the providers at the stroke center where recommendations were made related to stroke intervention. This program was very instrumental in addressing the management of stroke in the early symptomatic stages thus reducing complications.

Beth and her student decided to use the university's telemedicine platform, specifically tele-Conferencing, to provide a telehealth stroke education program to the elderly within one of the rural communities. In order to evaluate the effectiveness of the program, her student provided face-to-face education to one group of at-risk elderly individuals in the rural setting located 300 miles away, and then provided the same education to another group in the same area using telehealth. Her results showed that the telehealth education program was as effective as the face-to-face education (Schweickert and Rutledge 2011). This was further supported in other studies that showed telehealth education for those with cardiovascular disease and diabetes greatly improved the patient's satisfactions, knowledge, and the effectiveness of the care (Timmerberg *et al.* 2009; Winters and Winters 2007).

Based on these findings, the interprofessional group decided to include education for caregivers as part of the new technology-based model of care they were developing. The education could either be delivered through (1) an interactive medium such as videoconferencing, (2) a static medium in which written materials were posted, or (3) store and forward methods that included materials that were collected/developed for future use such as videos (Rutledge *et al.* 2011) (Figure 12.2). Using an interactive approach, they would provide opportunities for live chats and e-mail correspondence. Static materials would be provided in the form of written information such as brochures and fact sheets. Finally, they would provide educational content using videos that were recorded and stored for future use.

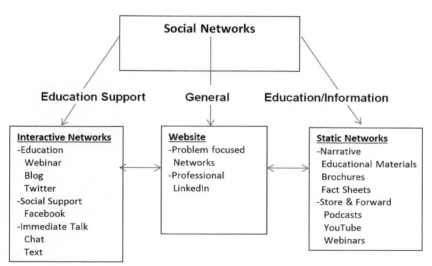

FIGURE 12.2. Tele-education.

TELEMONITORING

Beth had noticed that many of the frustrations she encountered with the caregivers were tied to a lack of sleep. Their sleep was often interrupted by the elderly individual wandering at night, worrying over how to best care for their loved one, and social isolation. These sleep disturbances contributed to a loss of work, increased illnesses, depression, and in the end, placement of the elderly individual in a nursing home. This decision was fraught with feelings of guilt and a sense of failure. Beth discussed her concerns with the interprofessional group. They decided that sleep hygiene should be part of the new model of care.

In exploring ways to incorporate sleep into the new model, a sleep actigraphy watch was identified. The watch had software that measured and recorded the quality of sleep, wakefulness, and night time movement. Sleep actigraphy home monitoring has become an essential tool within the last decade to assist practitioners in sleep research and sleep medicine. The use of sleep actigraphy monitoring has recently become available to the practitioner for home monitoring of their patients' sleep quality. This data can be downloaded weekly and sent to providers, enabling them to review their patient's sleep distantly from their offices. This type of information allows providers to tailor their sleep hygiene teaching and reinforce strategies that are working.

Sleep monitoring is not that different from other home monitoring that occurs between patients and their providers. Home monitoring involves audio, video, and other telecommunication technologies that run from real time or store and forward patient monitoring. Home monitoring systems include devices such as the actigraphy watch, blood pressure monitoring, scales for monitoring weight, glucose monitors, heart and respiratory monitoring, and home spirometry. Other home monitoring systems provide motion detection, allowing family and health professionals to monitor patients for falls and long periods of immobility. These medical home monitoring devices allow a home based nurse to transport the data, but they are designed simplistically enough for a patient or family member to key in or transmit the data to a healthcare provider for interpretation.

Home monitoring presents an alternative to managing individuals that are homebound or require close follow-up care. This type of monitoring assures the rapid transmission of clinical and physiologic data needed to determine timely changes to medical interventions. Home monitoring may prevent the deterioration of the patient's condition that ultimately results in increased office visits, emergency room trips, and costly admissions. Home monitoring has been used to replace follow-up appointments for patients with chronic conditions. Multiple studies have demonstrated that the immediate feedback by health professionals through home monitoring results in better disease control and medication compliance (Hansen *et al.* 2011; Browning *et al.* 2011).

INTERPROFESSIONAL COLLABORATION THROUGH TECHNOLOGY

Counseling

As the discussion continued, the group realized that each of the professions in the room had a vital role in addressing the needs of the caregivers and their loved ones. The clinical counselor began describing the issues she was recognizing with similar cases. First and foremost was the issue of caregiver burden and stress that often leads to symptoms of depression. Underlying these feelings is a sense of low self-efficacy. Further discussion enlightened the group on the technology approaches that could be used to assist the caregivers in addressing the psychosocial issues they were encountering.

Studies have shown that counseling through telehealth can be as effective as face-to-face counseling (McCoy *et al.* 2013; Wendell *et al.* 2011). Beth recounted the story of a psych-mental health nurse practitioner she had worked with that was counseling elderly patients in nursing homes via telehealth. Each patient in the nursing home that was on a psychotropic medication was required to have a counseling visit once a month. The nursing home was located in a rural area without access to a mental health provider. In order to meet the needs of the facility, the psych-mental health NP provided the counseling from her home 200 miles away. A nurse would take the patient to a private room and stay with the patient as they received the counseling via telehealth, thus enabling patients to have access to the needed services. Realizing that this was a need, the insurance providers paid for the visit in the same manner they would a face-to-face counseling visit.

Physical Therapy

The interprofessional group realized that there would also be a need for the input of the physical therapist. The physical therapist shared her experiences in working with children that had cerebral palsy. Following her physical therapy sessions using a treadmill, parents often reported that their children had an unusually good night's sleep and were much easier to manage. This in turn resulted in improvement in the parent's sleep as well as less stress. The physical therapist felt that videoconferencing with the homebound caregiver could improve their quality of sleep and stress. She would provide strategies that the caregivers could use for themselves as well as the care recipient. Not only would the physical therapy enhance both the caregiver's and the care recipient's sleep, it could also improve the caregivers' strength, thereby increasing their ability to transfer the care recipient safely. Rather than the traditional face-to-face physical therapy visit, this service could be provided using a home-based physical therapy videoconferencing platform. This would allow the caregiver to be assessed and treated more frequently and without disrupting their already busy schedule.

Studies have shown that videoconference-based physical therapy is a feasible method of delivery and monitoring for patients that require ongoing therapy or who are homebound. Elderly clients who have received only home-based videoconference physical therapy have demonstrated improvement in both strength and range of motion (Bernard *et al.* 2009). Physical therapy videoconferencing has also been successfully utilized for individuals with chronic pain. A recent study reported successful results with 2-hour videoconferencing sessions between a physical therapist and homebound patients with chronic pain. The sessions included relaxation training, posture correction, stretching and strengthening, aerobic exercises, and body mechanic training (Palyo *et al.* 2012). Videoconferencing provided the physical therapist the ability to not only assess strength and mobility, but to change therapy plans in a timely manner. As the number of individuals with chronic and multiple chronic illnesses increases, so should the use of home videoconferencing for physical therapy.

VIRTUAL HEALTHCARE NEIGHBORHOOD

Based on the information obtained by the interprofessional group, the decision was made to develop a Virtual Healthcare Neighborhood (VHN) (Figure 12.3). This neighborhood was provided through a secured firewall and password-protected website that was open to no more than eight caregivers per group. The small group size enabled the caregivers to develop close support networks with peers in similar situations. The VHN also provided the caregiver with peer and healthcare support from an interprofessional team consisting of Beth, the adult nurse practitioner, the clinical nurse specialist, the physical therapist, and the clinical counselor. The focus of the site was to improve the caregivers' sleep, their general self-efficacy, and to provide both healthcare and social support. Specifically, the VHN encompassed (1) asynchronous access to an allied healthcare team for questions and answers, (2) peer support through blogs, (3) the most current information related to self-care and caring for elderly with Alzheimer's and related dementias,

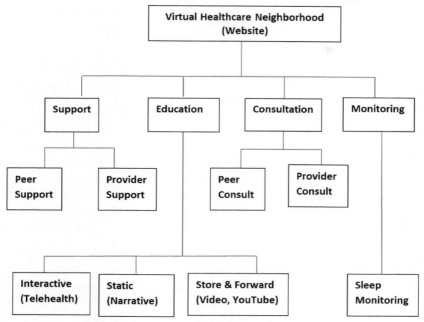

FIGURE 12.3. *Diagram of virtual healthcare neighborhood.*

(4) an online sleep hygiene programs that offered feedback on sleep quality via actigraphy, and (5) community resources.

The interprofessional group realized in the early design phase that the assistance from a computer scientist might be beneficial. The group invited a colleague from the university's computer science program to assist in the design and development of the VHN website. As the project was developed, the computer science team member suggested innovative ways to utilize personal tablets, how to incorporate interactive teaching modalities, and assisted with the development of the software for the actigraphy monitoring. Rather than spending unnecessary time trying to develop the website, the team was able to focus on the content. This truly represented an interprofessional effort that respected each other's strengths and abilities. Each member of the group was focused on the same outcome—to provide caregiver support through the use of technology.

CONCLUSION: TECHNOLOGY IN HEALTHCARE

The use of technology to provide services and treatment in healthcare has grown exponentially within the past 25 years (Luke et al.

2009). Many individuals are now relying on technology in an effort to take more responsibility for the care of themselves and for their loved ones. These technologies can provide opportunities and methods that can potentially improve healthcare disparities by providing access to healthcare information as well as timely interactions with healthcare professionals and social support groups regardless of whether the patient is being provided care locally or at a distance (Gibbons 2011).

In order for technology to truly make a difference in healthcare, there must be healthcare leaders and champions who incorporate these technologies into clinical practices and local communities. APNs are encouraged to lead the efforts to enhance the use of technologies in healthcare by not only mastering the technologies but also by collaborating with other healthcare providers in their use and application (IOM 2010). Due to their direct contact with patients and communities in both urban and rural areas, APNs are in a prime position to integrate healthcare technology into nursing care and develop innovative ways to improve patient care outcomes while addressing the pressing issues in healthcare today. This movement is supported by the National Organization of Nurse Practitioner Faculties (NONPF) NP Competencies that recommend that NP students be prepared in "technology and information literacy competencies," (2012). There is also strong support from other influential groups, such as the Institute of Medicine (IOM 2010) and the Health Resources and Services Administration (HRSA 2012) in fully incorporating technology into nursing practice and in working interprofessionally to provide patients access to care.

The role of APNs as leaders, change agents, and activists in the healthcare technology revolution can pay great dividends in addressing the healthcare crisis. This is especially important as the nation implements the Affordable Care Act. The APN can champion these new models of care as one potential solution to the nursing/provider shortage and misdistribution of healthcare services, thus improving care for the twenty-first century.

SUMMARY POINTS

- The use of telehealth improves communication, diagnosis, and treatment of patients.
- Telehealth platforms must be embraced by healthcare leaders who foster the improvement of patient care.
- APNs are on the forefront of incorporating telehealth into their practices to monitor patients and to provide quality patient care.

REFERENCES

Bernard, M., F. Janson, P.L. Flora, G.E.J. Faulkner, L. Meunier-Norman, and M. Fruhwirth. 2009. Videoconferencing-based physiotherapy and tele-assessment for homebound older adults: a pilot study. *Adaptation & Aging* (39–48). DOI:10.1080/01924780902718608

Browning, S.V., R.C. Clark, R.M. Poff, and D. Todd. 2011. Telehealth monitoring a smart investment for home care patients with heart failure? *Home Healthcare Nurse, 29*(6) (369–374).

Clifton, A., D. Goodall, S. Ban, and E. Birks. 2013. New perspectives on the contribution of digital technology and social media use to improve the mental wellbeing of children and young people: a state-of-the-art review. *Neonatal, Pediatric and Child Health Nursing, 16*(1) (19–26).

Gibbons, M.C. 2011. Use of information technology among racial and ethnic underserved communities. *Perspective in Health Information Management* (1–13).

Haney, T., K. Adams-Tufts. 2012. A pilot study using electronic communication in home healthcare: implications on parental well being and satisfaction caring for medically fragile children. *Home Healthcare Nurse, 30*(4) (216–224).

Hansen, D., A.L. Goldbeck, K. Lee, V. Noblitt, J. Pinsonneault, and J. Christner. 2011. Cost factors in implementing telemonitoring programs in rural home health agencies. *Home Healthcare Nurse, 29*(6) (375–382). Doi: 10.1097/NHH.0b013e31821b736f

Institute of Medicine. 2010. *The Future of Nursing—Leading Change, Advancing Health.* Retrieved http://books.nap.edu/openbook.php?record_id=12956&page=R1

Luke, R., P. Solomon, S. Baptiste, P. Hall, C. Orchard, E. Rukholm, and L. Carter. 2009. Online interprofessional health sciences education: from theory to practice. *Journal of Continuing Education in Health Professions. 29*(3) (161–167). doi: 10.1002/chp.20030

McCoy, M., L.R. Hjelmstad, and M. Stinson. (2013). The role of tele-mental health in therapy for couples in long-distance relationships. *Journal of Couple & Relationship Therapy, 12*(4) (339–358).

McDaniel, B.T., S.M. Coyne, and E.K. Holmes. 2012. New mothers and media use: Association between blogging, social networking, and maternal well-being. *Maternal Child Health Journal, 16* (1509–1517). doi: 10.1007/s10995-011-0918-2

Palyo, S.A., K.A. Schopmeyer, and J.R. McQuaid. 2012. Tele-pain management: Use of videoconferencing technology in the delivery of an integrated cognitive-behavioral and physical therapy group intervention. *Psychological Services, 9*(2) (200-202). doi 10.1037/a0025987

Phillips, B.C. 2010. Health care reform and the future of nursing and nurse practitioners. *Nurse Practitioners Business Owner Blog.* Retrieved. http://npbusiness.org/health-care-reform-future-nursing-nurse-practitioners/

Rutledge, C.M., M. Renaud, L. Shepherd, M. Bordelon, T. Haney, D. Gregory, and P. Ayers. 2011. Educating advanced practice nurses in using social media in rural healthcare. *International Journal of Nursing Education Scholarship, 8* (1) (1–14).

Schweickert, P. and C.M. Rutledge. 2011. Telehealth versus in-person stroke prevention education in elderly adults in Appalachian Virginia. *Telemedicine and e-Health,*
17(10) (1–5).

Social Media Today. 2013. *Social media in 2013: By the numbers.* Retrieved. http://
socialmediatoday.com/jonathan-bernstein/1894441/social-media-stats-facts-2013

Stanley, J.M., K.E. Werner, K. Apple. 2009. Positioning advanced practice nurses for
health care reform: Consensus on APRN reform, *Journal of Professional Nursing*
25(6) (340–348) doi: 10.1016/j.profnurs.2009.10.001

Timmerberg, B.D., J. Wurst, J. Patterson, R.J. Spaulding, and N.E. Belz. 2009. Feasibil-
ity of doing videoconferencing to provide diabetes education: A pilot study. *The Journal of Telemedicine and Telecare.* Retreived. 222.nbci.nl.nih.gov/pubmed/19246610

U.S. Department of Health and Human Services. 2008. *Addressing rural health care*
needs [testimony]. Morris, T: Author Retrieved. http://www.hhs.gov/asl/testi-
fy/2008/07/ 4312.html

U.S. Department of Health and Human Services. 2012. *The role of Telehealth in an*
evolving health care environment. Retrieved. http://www.hrsa.gov/ruralhealth/
about/telehealth

Wendell, M.L., D.F. Brossart, T.R. Elliott, C. McCord, and M.A. Diaz. 2011. Use of
technology to increase access to mental health services in a rural Texas community.
Family Community Health, 34(2) (134–140). doi: 10.1097/FCH.0b013e31820e0d99

Winters, J.M. and P.E. Winters. 2007. Videoconferencing and telehealth technologies
can provide a reliable approach to remote teaching without compromising quality.
Journal of Cardiovascular Nursing, 22 (51–57).

Using Technology to Improve Population-based Care

JOANNA D. SIKKEMA DNP, MSN, ANP-BC, FAHA, FPCNA
CHRISTINE C. HARSELL DNP, ANP-BC

Chapter 13 focuses on the skills needed to review data that impacts how evidence-based treatment for population based care is provided. A case study demonstrating the impact of health policy is presented.

Case Presentation

David is a family nurse practitioner based in a rural healthcare setting in the Midwest. He is the lone practitioner within a 500 mile radius. In general, his patient population is of a low socioeconomic status and is struggling to make a living. There are many generations living within each household in many cases and the responsibility of providership within the family is usually designated to the men of each family. Farm life is tough, especially in the brutal winter months which requires daily attendance to the animals, and in the summer which requires daily attendance to the crops as well as the animals. There is little time for illness to interfere with meeting the daily responsibilities of farm life. Therefore, David's patients often present with advanced disease and have often self-treated with a number of "home remedies."

David has learned to use his patient encounters as a chance to include important education, related to health promotion and disease prevention, to his patient population. He recently accessed data related to predicted influenza outbreaks in his community as well as immunization rates. These data are readily accessible on the CDC Flu Activity and Surveillance page. This year he is particularly concerned about a predicted influenza epidemic among his patient

155

population and the social and economic impact this will have upon the community. He is able to see in the clinic's EHR that nearly 30% of the clinic patients were treated for influenza last year. The immunization nurse at the clinic also reports that data from the state's immunization tracking database indicate that patients in their community are not likely to get immunized. The influenza vaccination rate was less than 25% for clinic patients last year. David would like to make increasing the rate of immunization a priority within the community and also efficiently provide patient education related to prevention and transmission of the flu within the households. The majority of David's patients are insured under Medicaid with limited economical resources, and David is acutely aware of the need to cover all practice expense to maintain a profit for the clinic.

In order to stay current with health and illness trends as well as current evidence, David uses a portion of his work week to review professional websites and journals online, as well as national databases for disease trends in his area. He also networks monthly with nurse practitioner colleagues and they share clinical updates and opportunities for enhancing rural practice. He is intrigued to learn that there are several grants available to APNs to provide enhanced influenza programming within their clinical practice. However, the funding is competitive and the need must be clearly defined. He is beginning to conduct a focused evidence-based data search to quantify the need for funding for his community health center flu prevention project.

David needs to compile several comprehensive state and national funding applications based on evidence-based practice to complete the various foundation grants which could possibly supply funding for such a project. He begins this process by beginning a data search utilizing a variety of available technologies to support his flu prevention programming. Once David has compiled the highest quality evidence to support his program, he synthesizes the body of evidence into a concise review of what is known about his topic. He is easily able to make the case for his flu prevention program and writes a successful grant.

David's flu prevention program includes two leading strategies: one that entails an immunization booth at the local weekly farmer's market, which is viewed as a social event in this rural farming community. The second initiative involves the distribution of "flupaks" which include I90 masks, antibacterial gel, soap, a small pack of tissues, a disposable paper bag, handiwipes, and information on the early signs and symptoms of influenza. The "flupaks" also included a card with websites and online resources for prevention, symptom recognition, and treatment. The local Girl Scout troop has volunteered to compile the "flupaks" as a community project and also help distribute them.

In order to promote his funded flu prevention program, David enlists the help of local organizations, media outlets, and several social media sites. He knows that the farmers will likely see the advertisements in the newspaper or on the local radio programming. He also knows that spouse and family members may be more apt to see advertisements at the local grocery store, in the school and church buildings, or on the clinic website. He enlists the help of key community members such as the pastors, teachers, and business owners to help spread the word. The clinic webpage highlights flu facts and promotes the "flupaks" as well as vaccination throughout flu season. David is interviewed by the local radio station about the project. The clinic also utilizes text message reminders for vaccination availability and appointments.

David's program is a success. Patient vaccination rates increased by nearly 50% from the previous year. Phone calls and visits related to flu symptoms decreased from precious years and the clinic even added patients from the extra advertising.

The local health department asks David if he will present his work and promising results at a regional conference. They believe that other rural community clinics may benefit from learning about this program and how to develop something similar.

ESSENTIAL CONTENT FOR USING TECHNOLOGY TO IMPROVE POPULATION-BASED CARE

The implementation of technology into nursing care is moving quickly at the bedside, home, and community at large. Historically, the implementation of healthcare technology was driven by cost-containment and organizational financial benefit. Furthermore, technology has transformed healthcare into providing high quality, evidence-based clinical care resulting in increased patient safety and satisfaction. This has been accomplished by increasing efficiencies and financial gain for those healthcare providers who are technologically engaged. Healthcare providers who are actively engaged in the understanding, evolution, utilization, and importance of technology in healthcare will be prepared for the healthcare systems of the future.

In order to stay current with health and illness trends as well as current evidence, David uses a portion of his work week to review professional websites and journals online, as well as national databases for disease trends in his area. He also networks on a monthly basis with nurse practitioner colleagues and they share clinical updates and opportunities for enhancing rural practice. He is intrigued to learn that there are several grants available to APNs to provide enhanced influenza programming within their clinical practice.

Legislative Mandates

Recent landmark healthcare reform legislation including the Health Information Technology for Economical and Clinical Health (HI-TECH) component of the American Recovery and Reinvestment Act (2009) and the Affordable Care Act (ACA) (2010) have significantly impacted the implementation of healthcare technology. This has been driven by the Electronic Health Record Incentive Program of the Centers for Medicare and Medicaid (CMS) providing incentives for eligible professional and hospitals to implement EHRs. These incentives are focused on improving care coordination, reducing duplicative tests and procedures, focusing on high-quality outcomes, and rewarding providers to keep patients healthier. This technology, being patient centered, supports the provider to better coordinate care, deliver the best practice, and reduce errors and readmissions (Murphy 2013).

The American Academy of Nursing Technology Drill Down Project (2007) funded by the Robert Wood Johnson Foundation identified that the areas of admission, discharge, and transfer (ADT); care coordination; care delivery; communication; documentation; medication; patient movement; and supplies and equipment all could benefit from greater integrated nurse friendly technology. This study identified that the use of barcodes, radio frequency identification (RFID) and robotic systems enhanced the safety and efficiency of delivering care. It concluded that the greatest impact of technology was written communication and data, followed by improvement in the safe delivery of care, system integration, supply chain, and oral communication. Technology was found to eliminate waste; alleviate some staffing and workload issues; assist in tracking staff, physicians, and patients; facilitate medication cycles; and improve the efficiency of the physical environment (Bolton 2008). The implementation of integrated technology networks in the healthcare system has transformed the delivery of health across departments, facilities, specialties, and providers by providing a more seamless environment for the integration of patient care processes.

The immunization nurse at the clinic also reports that data from the state's immunization tracking database indicate that patients in their community are not likely to get immunized. The influenza vaccination rate was less than 25% for clinic patients.

Technology and Nursing

Cipriano (2012) reported that the value of technology hinges on how it's used and whether it helps or hinders healthcare services. Technologies designed for and used by nurses at the point of care haven't been user friendly, and use of the Health Informational Technologies (HIT) platform mainly focused on medical practice. Consequently, nursing leadership has been slow to embrace technology to transform patient care. However, as more and more hospital systems change to accommodate the changes required by legislation, nurse leaders will have no choice but to meet the required regulations.

> He is able to see in the clinic's EHR that nearly 30% of the clinic patients were treated for influenza last year. David would like to make increasing the rate of immunization a priority within the community and also efficiently provide patient education related to prevention and transmission of the flu within the households he cares for. The majority of David's patients are insured under Medicaid with limited economical resources and David is acutely aware of the need to cover all practice expense to maintain a profit at the clinic.

Some of the emerging technologies that have impacted the delivery of nursing services have included the expansion of Internet services, mobile technologies, and healthcare social networks. For example, the use of telehealth and tele-education platforms have offered nurses and other providers remote access to highly specialized healthcare. Both healthcare professionals and patients can have face-to-face contact with each other to discuss their health needs. Often because of the availability of enhanced digital imagery, nurses, patients, and other providers can discuss interventions through telecommunication. Additionally, healthcare-specific social networks can help nurse practitioners deliver services, provide common social support to patients with similar disorders, and encourage patients to take an active role in their health.

> In order to promote his funded flu prevention program, David enlists the help of local organizations, media outlets, and several social media sites. He knows that the farmers will likely see the advertisements in the newspaper or on the local radio programming. He also knows that spouse and family members may be more apt to see advertisements at the local grocery store, in the school and church buildings, or on the clinic website. He enlists the help of key

community members such as the pastors, teachers, and business owners to help spread the word. The clinic webpage highlights flu facts and promotes the "flupaks" as well as vaccination throughout flu season. David is interviewed by the local radio station about the project. The clinic also utilizes text message reminders for vaccination availability and appointments.

Patient and Technology Demands

A recent survey found that 90% of patients want health information and education available online in order to help them better manage their own conditions. Eighty-three percent of patients surveyed wanted access to personal medical information online and 88% of those surveyed wanted to receive an e-mail reminder about preventive or follow up care (Accenture 2014).

The "flupaks" also included a card with websites and online resources for prevention, symptom recognition, and treatment.

As more and more healthcare technology platforms change, patients as well as providers will rapidly move from personal computers to mobile devices. The advent of mobile medical/healthcare computer applications (apps) has been estimated to range from 17,000–40,000 and continues to grow (Association of American Medical Colleges 2014).

TABLE 13.1. A Sampling of Patient/Consumer Apps (Lippman 2013).

Condition	Application
Anxiety	Breathe2Relax
Headache/Migraines	iHeadache
Medication OC Management	GoodRx MedMory myPill
Menopause	BioDesk myPause
Pain	WebMD Pain Coach
Sleep Problems	Sleep Diary
Voiding	Bladder Pal IP Voiding Diary
Weight Loss	Calorie Count Track to Lose It! MyFitness Pal

TABLE 13.2. Smart Phone Applications (Lippman 2013).

Function	Device
iHealth Body Analysis Scale	Body analysis
Withings BP Monitor	BP and heart rate
Masimo iSpO2	Oxygen saturation, pulse, perfusion index
Welch Allyn iExaminer	Fundoscopic examination
EyeNetra NETRA-G	Visual acuity
CellScope Oto	Ear drum visulaization
SpiroSmart Spirometer	Spirometry
AliveCor Heart Monitor	One-lead EKG
ThinkLabs ds32a + Stethoscope	Stethoscope
Mobisante mobiUS SP1 System	Ultrasound

A Pew Internet Study (2013) reported that seven out of ten U.S. adults track at least one health indicator for themselves or a loved one. Six in ten reported tracking weight, diet, or exercise and one in three said they track a medical problem such as headache, glucose level, or blood pressure (PEW 2014). The wide variety of medical applications range from recording a single lead electrocardiogram or a mobile device serving as an otoscope, to counting calories, monitoring exercise regimes, and providing medication information.

This technology explosion is enabling patients to assume greater responsibility for their healthcare and benefits providers with greater resources from which to make point-of-service evidence-based healthcare decisions. Table 13.2 lists some of the "Smart Phone Physical" (Lippman 2013) applications that are available.

Using Technology to Identify the Evidence

In the IOM's report, Crossing the Quality Chasm, the authors noted a vast difference between what we know about healthcare and what we do (IOM 2001). As a result of fostering a better scientific basis for what we do in clinical practice, the IOM report suggested that healthcare providers provide evidence for what works best in practice. Evidence-based practice (EBP) was endorsed as a way to provide quality patient care. Stevens suggested the following:

Clinical leaders have unprecedented opportunity to step forward to transform healthcare from a systems perspective, focusing on EBP for clinical effectiveness, patient engagement, and patient safety (2013).

TABLE 13.3. Patient Population, Intervention, Comparison, Outcome and Time (PICOT) (Melnyk 2010).

Letter	Clinical Question	Case Study
P	Patient population of interest	Rural families/Medicaid patients
I	Intervention or area of interest	Seasonal influenza program
C	Comparison intervention or group	No influenza program
O	Outcome	Increased vaccination rate
T	Time	3–6 months

The basic principles of EBP include combining the highest quality, current evidence, clinical expertise, and patient preference into care. Organizations must create a culture of EBP at all levels. It is vital to have leaders who value inquiry and questions about practices, policies, and decisions.

Utilizing supportive evidence to provide the background data for an innovative project is critical to justify funding and assure quality healthcare. With the advent of the Internet and current technology, we can view, review, and compile a wealth of information that can be personalized to a specific population. However, this information needs to be reviewed in an organized and relevant manner in order to be most effective. Utilizing critical terminology and key words can be a major challenge when faced with reviewing the evidence, especially when applying for funding, where relevance, brevity, and appropriateness are essential. Understanding how to best utilize the technology of electronic databases in an organized manner can assure a focused search of relevant information.

Melnyk and colleagues (2010) suggested using a systematic format known as population, intervention, comparison, outcome, and time (PICOT) to streamline database searches so as to best focus on the clinical question. Individuals who have used the PICOT method to organize and review databases have found it to be one method to review current or past clinical interventions.

FREQUENTLY USED HEALTHCARE DATABASES

There is a wide variety of information available to help to answer a clinical question and to develop the best evidence practice review. The main sources of information for addressing a clinical question include primary, secondary, tertiary, and gray sources. Primary sources consist of evidence from single, original studies related to a topic. Secondary literature provides commentary or discussion of primary literature such as a systematic review. Tertiary sources provide a collection of primary and secondary sources such as an encyclopedia or guideline. Finally, gray literature consists of works that may be available but are not necessarily published such as conference proceedings, white paper statements, dissertations, or theses.

An evidence hierarchy is a useful tool to begin to search a database and answer a clinical question. When viewing an evidence hierarchy, the "highest" level of evidence to answer a clinical question is a systematic review, followed by a primary literature review. Tertiary and gray literature would only be used after primary and secondary sources have been developed to ensure an exhaustive search of available literature on the topic. Figure 13.1 is an example of an evidence hierarchy.

Often times, a review of existing evidence related to your topic may already exist. A systematic review is a summary of research evidence that follows a clear set of guidelines for searching, assessing, and synthesizing the available evidence on a topic (Hemingway and Brerton 2009). If a high quality systematic review is available on your topic, it is considered the highest possible level of evidence you can use. Systematic reviews can be located in a variety of places however; the Cochrane Collaboration is 1 the most widely known available source (www.cochrane.org).

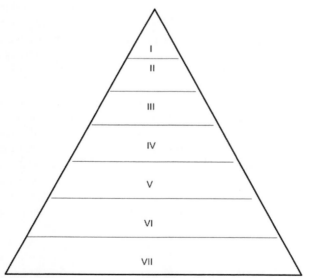

FIGURE 13.1. *Example of an evidence hierarchy. Level I: Systematic reviews or meta-analysis; Level II: Randomized control trials; Level III: Control trial without randomization; Level IV: Cohort or case control study; Level V: Systematic review of qualitative studies; Level VI: Qualitative study; Level VII: Expert opinion (Stillwell et al. 2010).*

If no systematic review is available, a search of primary literature should be conducted. Primary literature is evidence from single, original studies related to a topic. The most important of the primary databases for searches related to healthcare and nursing include PubMed and the Cumulative Index to Nursing and Allied Health (CINAHL).

PubMed is a site maintained by the U.S. National Library of Medicine National Institutes of Health. It contains over 23 million citations related to published medical and health research (http://www.ncbi.nlm.nih.gov/pubmed). CINAHL contains indexed citations, journals, and publications from nursing, biomedicine, health sciences, and other allied health professions (http://www.ebscohost.com/biomedical-libraries/the-cinahl-database)

> David needs to compile several comprehensive state and national funding applications based on evidence based practice to complete the various foundation grants which could possibly supply funding for such a project. He begins this process, by beginning a data search utilizing a variety of available technologies to support his flu prevention programming.

INCORPORATING STATE AND NATIONAL DATA

Advancing technology and increasing access to Internet resources has changed not only how providers access information and provide care, but it has had a profound effect on a patients' knowledge level and expectations about their care. There are a variety of resources to which patients and providers have access.

> David has learned to use his patient encounters as a chance to include important education, related to health promotion and disease prevention, to his patient population. He recently accessed data related to predicted influenza outbreaks in his community as well as immunization rates. These data are readily accessible on the CDC Flu Activity and Surveillance page. This year he is particularly concerned about a predicted influenza epidemic among his patient population and the social and economic impact this will have upon the community.

Table 13.4 provides a summary of some of the resources that nurse leaders and their patients may find useful in answering questions about a patient's health and well-being. Other places to access data related to specific topics include national professional organizations such as the American Nurses Association, http://www.nursingworld.org/, or edu-

TABLE 13.4. *Official State and National Databases to Access Healthcare Information for Patients and Healthcare Professionals.*

Name of Agency	Official Website	Overview of Available Information
U.S. Department of Health and Human Services (HHS)	http://www.hhs.gov/	The HHS strives to "help provide the building blocks that Americans need to live healthy, successful lives," (HHS 2013). There are multiple divisions of the HHS that each help to meets its mission at the national and state levels including the Centers for Disease Control and Prevention (CDC), Agency for Healthcare Research and Quality (AHRQ), National Institutes of Health (NIH), and Substance Abuse and Mental Health Services Administration (SAMHSA). The HHS website provides information about diseases and conditions as well as links to its many divisions.
Centers for Disease Control and Prevention (CDC)	http://www.cdc.gov/	The CDC is a federal government agency that works to "protect America from health, safety, and security threats both foreign and in the U.S." (CDC 2013). The site is filled with information about topics ranging from chronic disease, childhood illnesses, and major public health concerns like influenza and immunizations. There are resources available for all levels of consumers from school children and health consumers to healthcare providers.
Agency for Healthcare Research and Quality (AHRQ)	http://www.ahrq.gov/	The mission of the AHRQ is to "produce evidence to make healthcare safer, higher quality, more accessible, equitable, and affordable, and to work with the U.S. Department of Health and Human Services (HHS) and other partners to make sure that the evidence is understood and used," (AHRQ 2013). This site provides information for consumer, providers and systems in order to assist them in making sound evidence based decisions about healthcare.
National Institutes of Health (NIH)	http://www.nih.gov/	The NIH is the "nation's medical research agency," (NIH 2013). It supports research related to improving health, and the website provides a wealth of information about health, wellness, and disease processes.
Substance Abuse and Mental Health Services Administration (SAMHSA)	http://www.samhsa.gov/	SAMHSAs mission is to "reduce the impact of substance abuse and mental illness on America's communities," (SAMHSA 2013). This website provides information about substance abuse and mental illness for consumers as well as providers. It also provides data about treatment and services.
U.S. Census Data	http://www.census.gov/	The U.S. Census website provides information about the U.S. population and economy. Data about social, economic, housing, and demographic characteristics for the nation and by state can be accessed here.

cational organization like the American Heart Association, http://www.
heart.org/HEARTORG/.

TECHNOLOGY AND DISSEMINATION

Dissemination is simply spreading the word about what you have
done. Disseminating work about evidence-based practices is an integral
step in ensuring high quality healthcare. There are a variety of ways to
disseminate best practices. These include, but are not limited to, oral
presentations, poster presentations, meetings, publications, and media.

> The local health department asks David if he will present his
> work and promising findings at a regional conference. They believe
> that other rural community clinics may benefit from learning about
> this program and how to develop something similar.

No matter what the medium used, the presenter should have a clear
idea of who the audience is and what it is you want them to learn. When
doing presentations, PowerPoint slides or poster formats should be simple and interesting—avoiding any texts or graphics that overpower the
presentation. Submitting a manuscript requires considerable time and
effort. Finding a journal that matches the purpose of your manuscript
is a critical first step followed by multiple revisions and edits (Fineout-
Overholt *et al.* 2011).

Using media such as television, radio, and Internet sites is another
method to disseminate EBP findings. Many television or radio networks
have news segments related to health and wellness. In addition, local interest pieces such as David's immunization booth at the farmers market
or the Girl Scouts' involvement in making the "flupaks" can be called
to the televisions or radio producers' attention with a phone call or press
release. Similar principles apply here in terms of knowing your audience and having a clear and concise message. Even more recent is the
use of social media such as Twitter or Facebook to promote work or accomplishments. While these venues are becoming increasingly popular,
it is important to adhere to all policies associated with healthcare privacy. One helpful resource includes the American Nurses Association's
Principles for Social Networking and the Nurse (2011) that can be used
to guide one's action for the dissemination of data.

Nurses continue to be leaders in the healthcare technology industry both at the national and international level. Nurses are at the
frontline of providing safe, high quality, cost effective healthcare to
patient populations in a variety of settings. Use of these enhanced
by patient-focused technologies will continue to impact the quality

of patient care. Finally, the shifting healthcare system will require better coordination between the providers, insurers, and government agencies to provide quality care on a continuum with shared account-ability among all involved.

SUMMARY POINTS

- Legislative mandates such as the HITECH component of the American Recovery and Reinvestment Act (2009) and the Affordable Care Act (ACA) 2010 have significantly impacted the implementation of healthcare technology, particularly the EHR.
- The use of technology in healthcare encompasses electronic health records, evidence data bases, telecommunication between healthcare team members, patient access to information such as their health records, as well as coaching and education and the use of social media.
- Patients are increasingly embracing technology to access healthcare information and increase involvement in their care.
- The basic principles of evidence-based practice include combining the highest quality, current evidence, clinical expertise, and patient preference into healthcare. Increased access to technology can help increase EBP practices across organizations.
- It is vital to have leaders who value inquiry and questions about practices, policies, and decisions.
- Nurses are poised to take on leadership roles in the use of healthcare technologies and must continue to participate in evidence based practice, quality improvement, and dissemination of findings.

REFERENCES

Accenture. Retrieved February 28, 2014. http://www.accenture.com/us-en/Pages/insight-trends-health-what-future healthcare-technology-look-like.aspx

Agency for Healthcare Research and Quality. 2013. *AHRQ at a Glance*. Retrieved. http://www.ahrq.gov/about/index.html

American Nurses Association. 2011. Principles for social networking and the nurse. Silver Spring, MD.

Association of American Medical Colleges. 2012. *Explosive Growth in Health Care Apps Raises Oversight Questions*. Retrieved. https://www.aamc.org/newsroom/reporter/october2012/308516/health-care-apps.html

Bolton, L.B., C. Gassert, and P. Cipriano. 2008. Smart technology enduring solutions: Technology solutions can make nursing care safer and more efficient. *Journal of Health Information Management. 22* (4) (24–30).

Centers for Disease Control and Prevention. 2013. Mission, Role and Pledge. Retrieved. http://www.cdc.gov/about/organization/mission.htm

Cipriano, P. 2013. Enabling the ordinary: More time to care. *American Nurse Today.* *8*(11) (582).

Fineout-Overholt, E., S.B. Stillwell, L. Gallagher-Ford, and B.M. Melnyk. 2011. Evaluating and disseminating the impact of an evidence based practice intervention: Show and tell. *American Journal of Nursing 111*(7) (56–59).

Lippman, H. 2013. How Apps are changing family medicine. *Clinician Review, 23*(9) (26–31).

Melnyk, B.M., E. Overholt-Fineout, S. Stillwell, and K. Williamson. 2010. The seven steps of evidence-based practice. *American Journal of Nursing 110*(1) (51–53).

Murphy, J. 2013. Progress report: Electronic health records and HIT in the United States. *American Nurse Today 8*(11) (10–11).

National Institutes of Health. 2013. *About NIH.* Retrieved. http://www.nih.gov/about/

Pew Research Internet Project. Retrieved March 6, 2014. http://www.pewinternet. org/2012/11/08/mobile-health-2012/

Stillwell, S.B., E. Fineout-Overholt, B.M. Melnyk, and K.W. Williamson. 2010. Searching for evidence: Strategies to help you conduct a successful search. *American Journal of Nursing 110*(5) (41–47).

Substance Abuse and Mental Health Services Administration. 2013. *About Us.* Retrieved. http://beta.samhsa.gov/about-us

U.S. Department of Health and Human Services. 2013. *About HHS.* Retrieved. http://www.hhs.gov/about/

Interprofessional Healthcare Delivery

MARIDEE SHOGREN DNP, CNM

The intent of Chapter 14 is to address the concepts associated with interprofessional healthcare delivery models. An interprofessional model of clinical practice is explored.

Case Presentation

Elisabeth graduated from a baccalaureate program in nursing and returned to her rural hometown community to practice as a registered nurse at the local healthcare center. The healthcare center consisted of a 15 bed critical access hospital with emergency room and ambulance services, a medical clinic, and a 50-bed nursing home. The hospital also provided obstetric (OB) care for low-risk patients; approximately 30 families give birth in the hospital each year. Home healthcare services are affiliated with the center. The healthcare center is staffed by two family practice physicians, RNs, LPNs, and full-time laboratory personnel. Outreach support is provided several times a week and allows occupational therapy, physical therapy, speech therapy, and mental health professionals to work in the healthcare center to meet patient needs. Referrals for complex healthcare needs and specialty conditions are accommodated through a larger healthcare system located approximately 70 miles away from the community.

During her first 5 years as an RN, Elisabeth's roles changed daily as she found herself working in all aspects of the center caring for patients across the lifespan. Occasionally, she would pick up time in the nursing home and the clinic. As her experience and confidence grew, she developed strong working relationships with the

169

other healthcare providers and felt like everyone was part of a collaborative team.

While in her 6th year of nursing, Elisabeth was approached by one of the physicians who asked if she would be interested in returning to school to become an APN to help meet the growing healthcare demands of the community. The healthcare center was willing to support her tuition if Elisabeth would return to the center to practice for at least three years after graduation. Elisabeth agreed and entered a dual master's program to become a family nurse practitioner (FNP) and a certified nurse midwife (CNM).

During her graduate programs, Elisabeth often reflected on how much training had changed from her undergraduate education where she sat in a classroom with her peers. Enrolling in a graduate hybrid program allowed her to combine online classes with intermittent on-campus visits so that she could continue to live in her hometown and still work occasionally at the healthcare center. She noted how different this education was from a traditional program and at times missed the connection to classmates, shared hands-on experiences, and daily contact with professors. However, once her clinical experiences began, she felt more immersed in her educational experiences.

One of the clinical courses Elisabeth was required to take was an interprofessional healthcare course. This course was combined with students in physical therapy, occupational therapy, medicine, and clinical counseling. Students would "meet" online to discuss the benefits of interprofessional education (IPE) and collaborative practice. During their on-campus experiences, they would participate in group simulation and debriefing exercises that incorporated team leadership training, communication, and role development exercises. Elisabeth loved these experiences and looked forward to working as an APN in collaborative practice with her physician colleagues and outreach partners.

Upon graduation, Elisabeth returned to her hometown healthcare center as a full-time APN. She was welcomed back very enthusiastically and was given her own office and one staff nurse to work with her every day. Soon she found her schedules full of patients and shared OB calls. She had clinic staff meetings once every month and met with the on-call physician briefly for a "hand-off discussion" prior to taking over call once every weekday and every third weekend in the schedule. However, it seemed that the collaborative experience she had been looking forward to was nowhere to be found. Elisabeth often felt very alone in her practice as the only APN but also felt she lacked a mentor for her new role. She immediately encountered complex patient situations that were difficult to handle due to her inexperience. The physicians did not respond well to questions common for a new practitioner and often indicated that because she had been an employee of the healthcare center for so long she should "know how things work." She had difficulty referring patients for outreach services and was discouraged to find that patients often alternated visits with all providers which led to duplication of services, lack of continuity, and ultimately less than optimal patient outcomes. As her confidence decreased, she wondered if this was "just how it worked in real practice" or if there was truly a way to incorporate the IPE concepts she had learned about in school.

After practicing for 4 months with little improvement, Elisabeth contacted one of her colleagues from graduate school. This new FNP was practicing in another rural setting in a nearby state. In previous correspondence, her colleague had shared that she was enjoying her work and not experiencing the same issues as Elisabeth. They discussed differences between their practices and together created a plan that Elisabeth could bring to her colleagues to implement more collaborative teamwork and increase personal satisfaction in her role.

About 6 months after beginning her new job, Elisabeth was scheduled to meet with the two physicians to have her first formal evaluation. She had requested extra time so that she could adequately discuss her concerns. When the meeting began the physicians stated that they felt Elisabeth was doing very well in her role, that they detected no real problems, and suggested another meeting at the end of her first year.

Elisabeth had come to this meeting prepared, however. She had outlined her strategy and began by highlighting some of the positive aspects of the practice. She then listed some of the barriers she felt were presently impacting effective collaborative functioning of the new team and the items she felt would enable a more interprofessional approach to their patient care and improve patient outcomes. Finally, she suggested a full team meeting to introduce these collaborative ideas to the RNs, ancillary hospital and clinic staff, and the outreach professionals within the healthcare system.

The physicians listened and noted they had always been the leaders in the practice and felt comfortable with working independently. They were surprised at Elisabeth's observations. They admitted that while their education did not stress an interprofessional approach, they felt as if they had been working with the entire team in a collaborative manner because they had been referring to other providers and they had broadened their team to include an APRN. They appreciated the materials that Elisabeth had shared along with a description of the concepts she had learned in school and were open to more education in this area. Together they developed a 1 day, all staff meeting to take place in next few months. The meeting would introduce the interprofessional competency domains and include time for staff to share ideas through an interactive case study that would introduce interprofessional concepts to the healthcare team.

The initial meeting went very well and positive feedback was received by all participants. Upon its conclusion, plans were made to incorporate interprofessional simulation exercises and to hold team meetings three times a year to reinforce team collaboration. Elisabeth took on the leadership role for organizing the first of these future meetings. The group agreed to rotate leaders for the following two meetings of the year to share responsibilities. In addition, the group participated in ongoing continuing education classes that strengthened their own professional skills as well as improved their application of IP concepts.

ESSENTIAL CONCEPTS OF INTERPROFESSIONAL HEALTHCARE

Even though the concept of interprofessional healthcare is not new, there has been an explosion in the literature regarding the necessity for the implementation of IPE collaboration in clinical practice. IPE has been identified as "a necessary precursor to effective team functioning and quality care" (Disch 2013). The end goal of IPE is to build a better patient-centered healthcare system (IECEP 2011). As a result, more institutions of higher learning are including IP undergraduate and graduate courses in healthcare curriculums.

One of the clinical courses Elisabeth was required to take was an interprofessional healthcare course. This course was combined with students in physical therapy, occupational therapy, medicine, and clinical counseling. Students would "meet" online to discuss the benefits of IPE and collaborative practice. During their on-campus experiences, they would participate in group simulation and debriefing exercises that incorporated team leadership training, communication, and role development exercises. Elizabeth loved these experiences and looked forward to working as an APN in collaborative practice with her physician colleagues and outreach partners.

"Interprofessional education occurs when students from two or more professions learn about, from, and with each other to enable effective collaboration and improve health outcomes," (WHO 2010).

Interprofessional Models for Healthcare Education

There are several different frameworks guiding IPE. The World Health Organization's *Framework for Action on Interprofessional Education and Collaborative Practice* (2010) offers strategies for health policy-makers to implement IPE and collaborative practice. It includes the identification of institutional, working culture, and environmental mechanisms to introduce and execute collaborative practice throughout the world's healthcare system. A second framework, the *Interprofessional Education for Collaborative Patient-centered Practice: An Evolving framework* (D'Amour and Oandasan 2005), highlights the interdependence between IPE and collaborative practice. The framework demonstrates that IPE, through teaching and learning at pre- and post-licensure levels, enhances learner outcomes, thus promoting collaborative practice and enhancing patient outcomes. The competencies related to interdependency on the knowledge and skills learned through IPE directly impacts and improves patient outcomes.

Finally, the Commission on Education of Health Professionals for the 21st Century prepared a framework that redesigned the education of health professionals focusing on population health needs and improving the performance of health systems to meet these needs. The Commission called for a global social movement to integrate a public health approach to the education of healthcare providers. The framework suggests the use of nonhierarchical relationships and a multiprofessional approach to healthcare (Frenk *et al.* 2010).

Competencies for Interprofessional Education

After reviewing previously identified IP competencies in education and several IP frameworks, the Interprofessional Education Collaborative Expert Panel (IECEP) released its *Core Competencies for Interprofessional Collaborative Practice* (IECEP 2011). Six national associations of health professions schools served on the expert panel. These included nursing, osteopathy, pharmacy, dentistry, medicine, and public health. As a result, the following recommendations were supported to integrate four overall IP competency domains into all health professional curriculums: (1) values/ethics for interprofessional practice, (2) roles/responsibilities, (3) interprofessional communication, and (4) teams and teamwork. Today, these health professions have integrated

IP learning strategies and competencies in their respective educational programs.

Institutions can use the competency domains to guide integration of the interprofessional concepts into individual learning objectives and activities. The teaching methods include different interactive learning technologies like simulation, case study discussions, and community-based service projects that model real world collaborative practice for students. Students are expected to demonstrate these competencies during their clinical rotations. Ultimately, the goal is to use these skills in future clinical practice as leaders in healthcare systems who seek to improve patient care through effective patient outcomes.

TRANSITION FROM INTERPROFESSIONAL EDUCATION TO INTERPROFESSIONAL PRACTICE

While health professions continue to make curriculum changes that enhance IPE, there is ongoing controversy surrounding the traditional health core competencies. Often, educators are reluctant to embrace new trends without data that demonstrates that the new trends impact student outcomes. Unfortunately, most health professionals continue to be primarily educated within their own discipline. This is necessary to assure common experiences, values, and training of professional skills (Hall 2005). In an attempt to enhance education, IP concepts have been introduced into newer health education programs to blend these discipline-specific skills with more of a multidisciplinary approach to patient care. However, the addition of one or two interprofessional courses and placing a variety of healthcare professionals on a teaching team doesn't mean that they will automatically apply the knowledge and skills necessary to work together effectively and assure translation of these concepts (MacNaughton *et al.* 2013).

Elisabeth often felt very alone in her practice as the only APN but also felt she clacked a mentor for her new role. She immediately encountered complex patient situations that were difficult to handle due to her inexperience. The physicians did not respond well to questions common for a new practitioner and often indicated that because she had been an employee of the healthcare center for so long she should "know how things work." She had difficulty referring patients for outreach services, and was discouraged to find that patients often alternated visits with all providers which led to duplication of services, lack of continuity, and ultimately less than optimal patient outcomes.

In Elisabeth's scenario, the other providers may have actually felt that they were working as a collaborative healthcare team. However, in reality, they were independently functioning and not collaboratively sharing information needed to review the overall patient outcomes of the clinical practice.

> The physicians listened and noted they had always been the leaders in the practice and felt comfortable with working independently. They were surprised at Elisabeth's observations. They admitted that while their education did not stress an interprofessional approach, they felt as if they had been working with the entire team in a collaborative manner because they had been referring to other providers and they had broadened their team to include an APN.

Responsibilities were being shared at the healthcare center; although the physicians maintained primary leadership roles, provider options had been expanded for their patients by bringing in an APN, and they had worked together for several years prior to Elisabeth's role change. There was a perception that the work setting was comfortable for all providers because of their past shared experiences. In addition, this healthcare center had a long-standing relationship with several outreach health professionals from disciplines other than nursing and medicine. However, to Elisabeth it was clear that there was more independent practice among multiple providers than a true interprofessional model of healthcare delivery.

When interprofessional collaboration is effective, there is a shared understanding of each other's roles and responsibilities (Hall 2005). The team is structured so that the goal becomes shared decision-making with each professional contributing knowledge, expertise, and problem-solving skills. This collective identity is counter intuitive to many professions where independent decision making and autonomy are valued in their discipline (Golec-Harper and Clifford 2013). Accountability for one's actions enhances the patient's care since treatment options are discussed and the focus is on the patient and the best possible clinical care.

Models of care are evolving to help professionals blend IP concepts into high quality, effective patient care. One example used over the past decade is the Chronic Care Model (CCM) which was "designed to build on the interrelationships between six evidence-based elements that lead to improved clinical quality," (Coleman *et al.* 2009). This framework was initially used to guide quality improvement and improve interprofessional delivery in chronic care but has since been applied in many other primary care settings (Wagner *et al.* 2001). The model identifies six domains that contribute to effective interprofessional collaboration between healthcare providers and patients: (1) self-management support which focuses on helping patients and their families manage their own illnesses and emphasizes patient responsibility, (2) clinical information systems that support practice guidelines and patient care planning as well as identify subpopulations for care and monitor provider and system performance, (3) decision support that uses evidence-based resources to improve provider knowledge and skill, thus facilitating evidence-based clinical care, (4) delivery system redesign which helps define the division of labor with the team and facilitates planned patient visits so that one visit may include time with several team members, (5) healthcare organization that aims to bring interventions to a wider organization level, and (6) use of outside community resources. Application of these domains supports a more systematic approach to team collaboration, coordination of services, and a client-centered focus in primary care delivery (Hung *et al.* 2007; Stans *et al.* 2013).

A second clinical practice model that has been used to demonstrate interprofessional practice is the Clinical Practice Model (CPM) Framework (Westmoreland 2000) which guides practice and organizational culture transformation and supports integrated interdisciplinary practice at the point of care. This professional practice framework originated in nursing. The model incorporates systems thinking and continuous learning with six core beliefs that address (1) safe, individualized, holistic healthcare, (2) a healthy culture, (3) continuous learning, diverse thinking, and evidence-based practice, (4) partnerships to plan, coordinate, integrate, deliver, and evaluate healthcare, (5) personal accountability to communicate and integrate contributions to healthcare, and (6) quality is achieved from a shared purpose, vision, values, and healthy relationships. It also adopts the use of tools, resources, and clinical practice guidelines to support interprofessional practice. (Westmoreland *et al.* 2000; Wesorick and Doebbeling 2011). Using a practice model to guide interprofessional practice may lead to success, but there are barriers that must be identified in order for successful implementation.

Barriers That Impact Interprofessional Practice

Barriers to collaborative interprofessional practice are not difficult to identify. Status within the social order of health professionals, socialization and cultural, and educational and gender differences can all be barriers to team building and successful functioning (Ash and Miller 2014; Hall 2005; Whitehead 2007). Often, there is a misunderstanding or miscommunication about each professional's scope of practice or unfamiliarity of each profession's vocabulary and problem-solving skills. Territorial boundaries are frequently evident within group practices. Additionally, the structure of the healthcare system that rewards specialty practice may have contributed to the fragmentation or respect among healthcare professionals. When healthcare providers are deeply immersed in their own professional group, they may find fewer opportunities to engage with other disciplines and professions. The current payment systems are not structured to reward interprofessional collaboration and therefore do not provide an incentive for teams to work together (Ash and Miller 2014). Fee-for-service models and relative-value units may impede providers', especially physicians', participation in value-focused healthcare. These newer systems may not accurately reimburse or reward team-based activities, systems of care, population care, or creative and innovative measures to improve patient outcomes (Stecker and Schroeder 2013).

Issues associated with heavy workloads can easily lead to the time necessary to establish a collaborative team. Workforce limitations, an absence or fragmentation of services, and a lack of value for other professionals are equally prohibitive to effective collaboration (Parker *et al.* 2013). Even fatigue, stress, and team member turnover can all upset the balance of interprofessional practice (Hall 2005). Perhaps restructuring the number of patients a provider is responsible for as well as incentives that promote collaboration among the health disciplines would provide the needed support to increase collaborative practices.

Catalysts to Successful Collaborative Interprofessional Practice

Although there are barriers for interprofessional practice, most can be overcome if healthcare teams are encouraged to work together to provide effective patient-centered outcomes. Healthcare teams that want to develop collaborative practices must first develop a shared vision of how to work together and how to improve patient or population outcomes. This cements a community practice of team members with shared interests, engagement in information sharing activities, and the development of shared resources (Weiss *et al.* 2014).

Another catalyst to interprofessional practice is reciprocal trust. Mutual respect and trust are foundational to successful IP relationships that embrace cultural diversity and support individual differences in collaborative care (IECEP 2011). Team members must understand that trust takes time to develop. It is created through the demonstration of individual vulnerability and a willingness to give up control at times. It is enhanced through a culture of safe, open communication, face-to-face meetings, and team building workshops. When face-to-face meetings aren't a possibility, virtual trust may be created and is realistic with today's technology. Interestingly, meeting in person is thought to form trust through benevolence, but virtual trust development relies more on belief in team members' abilities and performance in the work place. Virtual team meetings using online communication can be enhanced with video conferencing (Ash and Miller 2014).

Trust may likewise be enhanced by the identification and understanding of each other's roles, scope of practice, and area of expertise. This can potentially alleviate future conflict by helping prevent role overlap on the team and serve as a means to prevent missed tasks in the plan of care (Ash and Miller 2014). Role discussion is a great place to recognize that professionals will differ in their levels of expertise.

The team will often consist of novices to experts, and these levels may fluctuate during the time the team is together. As more team members grow into experts there is a risk that independent practice will become the norm, but this should not be allowed to hurt team function; rather it should enhance synergy within the team. In high doses, independence without shared roles can stifle collaboration, but, "autonomy can be complementary to team work and enhance collaboration by promoting collegial relationships between team members," (MacNaughton 2013).

Autonomous providers are often respected for their knowledge and expertise and can provide crucial mentoring to the team. They may offer leadership skills as well. It is important to remember that the role of the leader does not have to be the physician on the team. With the realization that all healthcare professionals need to work to the top of their licenses and scope of practice, it should be understood team leadership will change according to the situation at hand and who is best suited for the role at that time. Different team members may need to lead different aspects of patient care to produce the most cost-effective and positive solutions. Working effectively will require that members become comfortable with relinquishing some professional autonomy to achieve better outcomes (IECEP 2011).

Finally, a catalyst to further develop collaborative practice may be found in improving interprofessional continuing education options. Because of the growing emphasis on team-centered care and the benefits of effective communication within a team, continuing education opportunities are being developed to meet these demands (Balmer 2013). This is especially important for healthcare professionals who were educated at a time when interprofessional concepts weren't as readily noted in curriculums. However, it is equally important for newer professionals who have been introduced to interprofessional concepts but now need continuous reinforcement of how to implement these ideas into their practices to keep the momentum going.

The initial meeting went very well and positive feedback was received by all participants. Upon its conclusion, plans were made to incorporate interprofessional simulation exercises and to hold team meetings three times a year to reinforce team collaboration. Elisabeth took on the leadership role for organizing the first of these future meetings. The group agreed to rotate leaders for the following two meetings of the year to share responsibilities. In addition, the group participated in ongoing continuing education classes that strengthened their own professional skills as well as improved their application of IP concepts.

There are many stakeholders who hold an interest in the improvement of our healthcare system. All health professionals hold an obligation to stay updated on current standards of care, communication and team-based strategies for improving patient outcomes, and systems-thinking approaches to improve population health and practice environments. Practicing health professionals must recognize that IPE is simply a part of their commitment to lifelong learning (Golec-Harper and Clifford 2013). The current healthcare delivery system is going through continuous reform that challenges healthcare professionals to imagine new ways of providing comprehensive, patient-centered care (Ash and Miller 2014). Advancements in continuing education options will certainly facilitate these needed improvements.

ADVANTAGES OF INTERPROFESSIONAL PRACTICE AND FUTURE DIRECTIONS

Reduced healthcare errors, decreased length of stays, improved patient and population health, and higher rates of patient satisfaction are just a few of the ways that effective interprofessional practice has made a difference in healthcare (Ash and Miller 2014). If healthcare is going to continue to improve globally, academic leaders have a responsibility to provide resources for faculty development and to support implementation of IPE in all health profession curriculums. Efforts are needed to enhance collaborative learning opportunities for healthcare students from multiple disciplines, especially those in distance programs, so that students can learn together to work together. Assessment of interprofessional competencies will be crucial to on-going evaluation of the efficacy of this movement (IECEP 2011).

Secondly, healthcare providers must recognize the importance of integrating these IP concepts into patient care. APNs are well positioned to participate in and lead interprofessional teams in efforts to improve health outcomes. As more APNs and other professionals, like physical therapists and pharmacists, become doctorally educated and encouraged to practice at the top of their education and scope, these new providers will both collectively and independently step into leadership roles they have never been in before, bringing a new dimension of expertise to interprofessional collaboration (Ash and Miller 2014).

Finally, the undiscovered advantages of interprofessional practices can only be identified with continuous research and dissemination of knowledge. Healthcare providers must not only come together with each other but with policy makers, administrators, informatics specialists, and even business leaders to improve patient health and population outcomes. Application of evidence-based research in clinical practice has the ability to reform all systematic levels of healthcare. Interprofessional education, collaboration, and practice are vital components to a complete transformation of world-wide healthcare delivery.

SUMMARY POINTS

- IPE has become an essential element in the curriculums of health professionals across disciplines.
- The Interprofessional Education Collaborative identified four competency domains for IPE: Values/ethics, roles/responsibilities, communication, and teams/teamwork.
- IPE does not always transition into interprofessional practice. More work is needed to facilitate this process and remove barriers to collaborative practice.
- Models of care, like the Chronic Care Model and the Clinical Practice Model Framework, are evolving to help healthcare professionals blend IP concepts into effective care.
- Interprofessional collaboration leads to reduced healthcare errors, decreased length of stays, improved patient and population health, and higher rates of patient satisfaction.

REFERENCES

Ash, L. and C. Miller. 2014. Interprofessional collaboration for improving patient and population health. In M. Zaccagnini and K. White (Eds.). *The doctor of nursing practice essentials: A new model for advanced practice nursing* (217–256). Burlington, MA: Jones & Bartlett Learning.

Balmer, J. 2013. The transformation of continuing medical education (CME) in the United States. *Advances in Medical Education and Practice, 4* (171–182).

Coleman, K., B. Austin, C. Brach, and E. Wagner. 2009. Evidence on the chronic care model in the new millennium. *Health Affairs, 28* (1), 75–85. doi: 10.1377/hlthaff.28.1.75

D'Amour, D. and I. Oandasan. 2005. Interprofessionality as the field of interprofessional practice and interprofessional education: An emerging concept. *Journal of Interprofessional Care, 1* (8–20). doi: 10.1080/13561820500081604

Frenk, J., L. Chen, Z. Bhutta, J. Cohen, N. Crisp, N., et al. 2010.Health professionals for a new century: Transforming education to strengthen health systems in an interdependent world. *Lancet, 376* (1923–58). doi:10.1016/S0140-6736(10)61854-5

Golec-Harper, L. and J. Clifford. 2013. Simplicity: The ultimate sophistication of collaborative practice. *Newborn & Infant Nursing Reviews, 13* (124–136).

Hall, P. 2005. Interprofessional teamwork: Professional cultures as barriers. *Journal of Interprofessional Care, S1* (188–196). doi: 10.1080/13561820500081745

Hung, D., T. Rundall, A. Tallia, D. Cohen, H. Halpin, and B. Crabtree. 2007. Rethinking prevention in primary care: Applying the chronic care model to address health risk behaviors. *The Milbank Quarterly, 85*(1) (69–91).

Interprofessional Education Collaborative Expert Panel (IECEP). 2011. Core competencies for interprofessional collaborative practice: Report of an expert panel. Washington, D.C. Interprofessional Education Collaborative. Retrieved. http://www.aacn.nche.edu/education-resources/IPECReport.pdf

Macnaughton, K., S. Chreim, and L. Bourgeualt. 2013. Role construction and boundaries in interprofessional primary healthcare teams: A qualitative study. *BioMedical Centraol Services Resaerch, 13*(1) (1–13). doi: 10.1186/1472-6963-13-486

Parker, V., K. McNeil, I. Higgins, R. Mitchell, P. Paliadelis, M. Giles, and G. Parmenter. 2013. How health professionals conceive and construct interprofessional practice in rural settings: A qualitative study. *BMC Health Services Research, 13* (1–11).

Stans, S., J. Stevens, and A. Beurskens. 2013. Interprofessional practice in primary care: Development of a tailored process model. *Journal of Multidisciplinary Healthcare, 6* (139–147).

Stecker, E. and S. Schroeder. 2013. Adding value to relative-value units. *The New England Journal of Medicine, 369*(23) (2176–2179). doi: 10.1056/NEJMp1310583

Wagner, E., B. Austin, C. Davis, M. Hindmarsh, J. Schaefer, and A. Bonomi. 2001. Improving chronic illness care: Translating evidence into action. *Health Affairs, 20*(6) (64–78). doi: 10.1377/hlthaff.20.6.64

Weiss, D., F. Tilin, and M. Morgan. 2014. *The interprofessional health care team:Leadership and development.* Burlington, MA: Jones & Bartlett Learning.

Wesorick, B. and B. Doebbeling. 2011. Lessons from the field: The essential elements for point-of-care transformation. *Medical Care, 49*(12) (S49–S57).

Westmoreland, D., B. Wesorick, D. Hanson, and K. Wyngarden. 2000. Consensual validation of clinical practice model practice guidelines. *Journal of Nursing Care Quality, 14*(4) (16–27).

Whitehead, C. 2007. The doctor dilemma in interprofessional education and care: how and why will physicians collaborate? *Medical Education, 41*(10) (1010–1016). doi:10.1111/j.1365-2923.2007.02893.x

World Health Organization (WHO). 2010. *Framework for action on interprofessional education & collaborative practice.* Retrieved. http://whqlibdoc.who.int/hq/2010/WHO_HRH_HPN_10.3_eng.pdf

Improving Clinical Outcomes Through Interprofessional Population-Based Clinical Practice

LAUREL S. SHEPHERD PHD., RN

Chapter 15 exposes the APN to future ideas related to monitoring, accountability, and providing interprofessional, evidence-based clinical care. Topics include ideas associated with "safe" clinical care within future healthcare systems.

Case Presentation

An 86 year-old, frail woman with diabetes who was experiencing hyperglycemia visited the office of her local provider. A NP met with her and made the usual adjustments to her medications. However this visit was different since she not only met with the NP but talked with a number of others about exercise, diet, and blood glucose self-monitoring, and they discussed what support she would need to make changes in these areas as well. She went home, were she lives alone and independently, to adjust to these new recommendations.

Within a few weeks, a care manager, to whom the woman reported her daily blood glucose levels and other vital diabetes related information, called the woman. This information had been recorded in an online application that the care manager had been trained to use at the office. Based on these results, the NP made further changes to the woman's medications, and this process was repeated in a few weeks.

Most recently, the woman developed pneumonia and required hospitalization. Fortunately, she had been part of a transitional care program that coordinates her care among providers and delivery settings from home to hospital and back home again. She also is part of patient centered healthcare or medical home (PCMH).

Advanced practice roles have expanded to include multiple specialties, practice sites, and populations. These are described in the Consensus Model for APN: Licensure, Accreditation, Certification and Education (2008). APNs have expanded in numbers and capabilities over the past several decades as they are highly valued and an integral part of the healthcare system. APNs include certified registered nurse anesthetists, certified nurse-midwives, clinical nurse specialists, and certified nurse practitioners. Some of these roles, such a midwifery and nurse practitioner, are strongly rooted in the traditions of community health nurses in meeting the needs of underserved populations and communities. There has been controversy and support for the expanding roles of nurses. Many of the questions regarding the capability of nurses to expand their practice have been answered (Brown and Grimes 1995). The research has indicated repeatedly for over two decades that advanced practice nurses are viewed by the public as capable and highly satisfactory providers (Newhouse *et al.* 2011). The development of the APN role has been questioned by other providers citing a fear for patient safety and care quality. Research has shown that advanced practice nurses meet or exceed physician providers in quality, acceptance and satisfaction (Newhouse *et al.* 2011). The APN is an essential member or leader of a healthcare team in an integrated delivery model of care. The research supports the excellent outcomes of care provided by nurse practitioners individually and as part of interdisciplinary teams.

> Fortunately, she had been part of a transitional care program that coordinates her care among providers and delivery settings from home to hospital and back home again. She also is part of a PCMH.

The American Academy of Pediatrics developed the concept of a medical home four decades ago, however, its meaning has evolved. The PCMH is a team approach to primary care that involves better care coordination and information systems (including the EHR) and gives patients greater access to care and to their providers (including e-mail exchanges). The main focus of this model is that the patient is at the center of decision-making. The patient is involved in discussions with all healthcare providers about his or her overall care and the recommendations of each team member. Transitional care targets older adults with two or more risk factors, including a history of recent hospitalizations, multiple chronic conditions, and poor self-health ratings.

One example of a transitional care program is located at the University of Pennsylvania, Transitional Care Model (2012). This program has ten essential elements that integrate the role, functions, and accountability for each team member as the patient moves throughout the system. These include:

1. *The transitional care nurse*, a master's prepared nurse with advanced knowledge and skills in the care of this population, as the primary coordinator of care to assure continuity throughout acute episodes of care.
2. *In-hospital assessment*, collaboration with team members to reduce adverse events and prevent functional decline, and preparation and development of a streamlined, evidenced-based plan of care.
3. *Regular home visits* by the Transitional Care (TC) nurse with available, ongoing telephone support (seven days per week) through an average of two months post-discharge.
4. *Continuity of care* between hospital and primary care providers is facilitated by the TC nurse accompanying patients to first follow-up visit(s).
5. *Comprehensive, holistic focus* on each patient's goals and needs including the reason for the primary hospitalization as well as other complicating or coexisting health problems and risks.
6. *Active engagement* of patients and family caregivers with focus on meeting their goals.
7. *Emphasis on patients'* early identification and response to healthcare risks and symptoms to achieve longer-term positive outcomes and avoid adverse and untoward events that lead to readmissions.
8. *Multidisciplinary approach* that includes the patient, family caregivers, and healthcare providers as members of a team.
9. *Physician-nurse collaboration* across episodes of acute care.
10. *Communication* to, between, and among the patient, family caregivers, and healthcare providers.

Transitional care advocate, Mary D. Naylor PHD., RN, FAAN, a professor of gerontology and director of the New Courtland Center for Transitions and Health at the University of Pennsylvania states that the model includes more than discharge planning and care coordination. The role of the APN is to help the patient and family set goals during hospitalization, design a plan of care that addresses them, and coordinates various care providers and services.

The APN then visits the home within 48 hours of discharge and provides telephone and in-person support as often as needed for up to 3 months. Assessing and counseling patients and accompanying them to medical appointments is aimed at helping patients and caregivers to learn the early signs of an acute problem that might require immediate help and to better manage patients' healthcare. Also essential is ensuring the presence of a primary care provider. In three randomized controlled trials of Medicare beneficiaries with multiple chronic illnesses, use of the TCM lengthened the period between hospital discharge and readmission or death and resulted in a reduction in the number of rehospitalizations (Naylor 1994; Naylor et al. 1999, 2004). The average annual savings was $5,000 per patient. Until now, transitional care has not been covered by Medicare and private insurers. But the Affordable Care Act sets aside $500 million to fund pilot projects on transitional care services for "high-risk" Medicare beneficiaries (such as those with multiple chronic conditions and hospital readmissions) at certain hospitals and community organizations over a 5-year period.

ADVANCED PRACTICE NURSES PRODUCE QUALITY PATIENT OUTCOMES

There is abundant and consistent evidence that APNs provide high quality care in an expanding array of environments and populations. In a meta-analysis of 38 studies comparing patient outcomes, nurse practitioner, and physician managed patient outcomes, those cared for by nurse practitioners had greater adherence to recommendations, patient satisfaction, and resolution of pathological conditions (Brown and Grimes 1995). The care provided by nurse practitioners has been shown to be consistently equivalent to care provided by physicians in primary care settings. However, research indicates that nurse practitioners demonstrated more time with patients, more complete documentation, and better communication skills (Horrocks et al. 2002). A meta-analysis of 16 studies of outcomes of APNs and physicians concluded that measures of quality of care, health outcomes, resource utilization, and costs were equivalent (Lauret). These findings were further supported in a study in which 1,316 patients were randomly assigned to nurse practitioners or physicians for primary care. After 6 months, the ratings for health status, health service utilization, and patient satisfaction were the same for both groups. However, patients treated by nurse practitioners had lower diastolic blood pressure values (Mundinger 2000). These findings were consistent at a 2-year follow-up (Lenz 2004).

Brooten and her colleagues (2002) conducted a review of the results of seven randomized clinical trials with very low birth-weight infants; women with unplanned cesarean births, high risk pregnancies, and hysterectomy surgery; elders with cardiac medical and surgical diagnoses and common diagnostic related groups; and women with high risk pregnancies in which half of physician prenatal care was substituted with APN care. Results indicated that outcomes of care by advanced practice nurses were of high quality with excellent patient outcomes across populations, specialties, and practice settings (Brooten *et al.* 2002).

A systematic review of advance practice nurse outcomes from 1999 to 2008 concluded that NP outcomes are comparable to those of physicians. The outcomes included patient satisfaction, patient perceived health status, functional status, hospitalizations, ED visits, and biomarkers including blood glucose, serum lipids, and blood pressure (Newhouse 2011).

INTEGRATED MODELS OF CARE

The Affordable Care Act provides support for new emerging models, including nurse-led clinics and integrated delivery models. Many of these new models included an advanced practice nurse as a leader or coordinator of care. The federal government has recognized the essential role for nurses and has provided additional funding to test new models of care and to train additional advanced practice nurses to be part of these initiatives ($15 million for a small demonstration project that will support 10 nurse-managed clinics for 3 years; $30 million to cover educational expenses to train 600 nurse practitioners; and $200 million for a clinical training demonstration project designed to increase production of advanced-practice nurses, including nurse practitioners).

New models of integrated care provide comprehensive, patient-centered care using patient-centered healthcare homes and accountable care organizations.

These models include familiar themes to nurse providers, coordinated care, and health promotion.

Bradway *et al.* (2012) investigated a quality cost model for transitional care. The purpose of the study was to describe the development, testing, modification, and results of the quality cost model of APNs for transitional care. The model provides care to clients as they age and move within the components of the healthcare system. The APN has a vital role in the coordinating and in leading this effort. Findings indicated that APN intervention consistently resulted in improved patient outcomes and reduced healthcare costs. Groups with APN providers were rehospitalized for less time at less cost, reflecting early detection and intervention.

OUTCOMES OF PATIENT CARE WITH
INTERDISCIPLINARY TEAMS

The presence of APNs on health teams improves patient outcomes in differing delivery settings and populations. A cross sectional study of 46 practices was conducted to determine quality measures of adherence to American Diabetes Association guidelines. Those practices that included NP's performed better on these measures including measurement of glycosylated hemoglobin, lipids, and microalbumin levels (Ohman-Strickland 2008). Long-term care patients managed by teams that include APNs are less likely to have falls, urinary tract infections, and pressure sores. In addition, they demonstrate improved functional status and have more consistent control of their chronic conditions (Bajerjian 2008).

Interdisciplinary, high quality chronic care delivery has been shown to improve the experiences of patients, although the results of the different models have been mixed. A study was conducted to determine patients' experiences and care quality in chronic care. Providers and patients in 17 disease management programs were included, targeting patients with cardiovascular diseases, chronic obstructive pulmonary disease, heart failure, stroke, comorbidity, and eating disorders. Overall, care quality and patients' experiences with chronic illness care delivery significantly improved. After adjusting for patients' experiences with care delivery, age, educational level, marital status, gender, and mental and physical quality of life, analyses showed that the quality of chronic care delivery and changes in care delivery quality predicted patients' experiences with chronic care delivery at a second visit (Cramm). This research showed that high quality interdisciplinary care resulted in more positive experiences of patients with various chronic conditions. The purpose of this study was to describe barriers and facilitators to implementing a transitional care intervention for cognitively impaired older adults and their caregivers lead by APNs. APNs implemented individualized approaches and provided care that exceeded the type of care typically staffed, and reimbursed in the American healthcare system by applying a transitional care model, advanced clinical judgment, and doing whatever was necessary to prevent negative outcomes. Reimbursement reform as well as more formalized support systems and resources are necessary for APNs to consistently provide such care to patients and their caregivers during this vulnerable time of transition.

Boult, Leff, and Boyd (2013) evaluated the outcomes of the guided care model of comprehensive interdisciplinary care that included primary care-based management, transitional care, and support for self management and family care giving. This model included a registered nurse working with two to five physicians in a practice to provide 50–60 high risk patients with multiple morbidities with eight services: home-based assessments, evidence-base care planning, proactive monitoring, care coordination, transitional care, coaching, and access to community based services. There were 904 high-risk older patients in eight primary care practices participating. After a 32-month test of this model, functional health of the primary care patients did not significantly improve. However, patient ratings of quality of care were higher. Patients increased their access to telephone support but their use of home health declined. The authors suggest that these findings may be due to a defect in the guided model or a difference in application of the model among the eight primary care practices. The authors concluded that the guided care model with the RN and MDs did not lead to control of the use and costs of care. The model incorporates the use of the RN and not the APN. The model may have been more effective by the addition of the APN to the mixed delivery model.

SUMMARY POINTS

- The principles of advanced nursing practice are based on evidence associated with "best practice" guidelines.
- The APN is a vital leader or a complimentary member of an integrated health team.
- The APN focuses on the client or patient and the family caregivers as the center of all care models of delivery.
- APN practice in a collaborative practice model includes the ability to work with other healthcare professionals, to measure outcomes of care, and to redesign care delivery as needed to ensure quality.
- Advanced practice nurses select and design outcome measures that focus on the patient and the effectiveness of care meeting patient needs.

REFERENCES

Abdus, S. and T. Selden. 2013. Preventive services for adults: How have differences 36 across subgroups changed over the past decade? *Medical Care, 51*(11) (999–1007).

Bakerjian, D. 2008. Care of nursing home residents by advanced practice nurses: A review of the literature. *Research in Gerontological Nursing, 1*(3) (177–185).

Bodenheimer, T. and H. Hoangmai. 2010. Primary Care: Current Care: Current Problems and Proposed Solutions, *Health Affairs 29*, no. 5 (799–805).

Boult, C., B. Leff, and C. Boyd. 2013. A matched–pair cluster-randomized trial of guided care for high-risk older patients. *Journal of General Internal Medicine, 28*(5) (612–621).

Bradway, C., R. Trotta, M. Bixby, E. McPartland, M. Wollman, H. Kapustka, K. Mc-Cauley, and M. Naylor. 2012. *Gerontologist.* Jun 2012; *52*(3) (394–407).

Brown, S.A. and D.E. Grimes. 1995. A meta-analysis of nurse practitioners and nurse midwives in primary care. *Nursing Research, 44*(6) (332–9).

Ettner, S.L., J. Kotlerman, A. Abdelmonen, S., Vazirani, R.D. Hays, and M. Shapiro. 2006. An alternative approach to reducing the costs of patient care? A controlled trial of the multi-disciplinary doctor-nurse practitioner model. *Medical Decision Making, 26* (9–17).

Goodell, S., C. Dower, and E. O'Neill. 2011. *Primary Care Health Workforce in the United States*, Research Synthesis Report No. 22, Robert Wood Johnson Foundation.

Horrocks, S., E. Anderson, and C. Salisbury. 2002. Systematic review of whether nurse practitioners working in primary care can provide equivalent care to doctors. *British Medical Journal, 324* (819–823).

Institute of Medicine. 2011. *The Future of Nursing: Leading Change*, Advancing Health.

Jiang, B. and S. Jiang. 2013. Hospital cost and quality performance in relation to market forces: An examination of US Community hospitals in the "post managed care era". *International Journal of Health Care Finance and Economics, 13* (53–71).

Kaiser Family Foundation. 2011. *Improving Access to Adult Primary Care in Medicaid: Exploring the Potential Role of Nurse Practitioners and Physician Assistants.*

Kern, L., R. Kaushel, and S. Malhotra. 2013. Accuracy of electronically reported "meaningful use" clinical quality measures. *Annals of Internal Medicine, 158* (77–83).

Lenz, E.R., M.O. Mundinger, R.L. Kane, S.C. Hopkins, and S.X. Lin. 2004. Primary care outcomes in patients treated by nurse practitioners or physicians: Two-year follow-up. *Medical Care Research and Review. 61*(3) (332–351).

McDonald, M., B. Matesic., and D. Contopoulos-Ioannid. 2013. Patient safety targete at diagnostic errors. *Annals of Internal Medicine 158*(5) Part 2 (381–389).

Morrison, F., M. Schubina, and S. Goldgerg. 2013. Performance of primary care physicians and other providers on key process measures in the treatment of diabetes. *Diabetes Care 36*(6) (1147–1152).

Mundinger, M.O., R.L. Kane, E.R. Lenz, A.M. Totten, W.Y. Tsai, and P.D. Cleary. 2000. Primary care outcomes in patients treated by nurse practitioners or physicians: A randomized trial. *Journal of the American Medical Association, 283*(1) (59–68).

Newhouse, R., J. Stanik-Hutt, K. White, M. Johantgen, E. Bass, G. Zangaro, R. Wilson, *et al.* 2011. Advanced practice nurse outcomes 1999–2008: A systematic review. *Nursing Economics, 29*(5) (1–22).

Naylor, M. and E. Kurtzman. The Role of Nurse Practitioners in Reinventing Primary Care, *Health Affairs 29*, no. 5 (2010) (893–9).

Ohman-Strickland, P.A., A.J. Orzano, S.V. Hudson, L.I. Solberg, B. DiCiccio, Bloom, and D. O'Malley. 2008. Quality of diabetes care in family medicine practices: Influence of nurse practitioners and physician's assistants. *Annals of Family Medicine, 6*(1), (14–22).

Pohl, J., C. Hanson, J. Newland, and L. Cronenwett. 2010. Unleashing Nurse Practitioners' Potential to Deliver Primary Care and Lead Teams, *Health Affairs 29*, no. 5 (900-5).

Robert Wood Johnson Foundation. 2012. *Implementing the IOM Future of Nursing Report—Part III: How Nurse Are Solving Some of Primary Care's Most Pressing Challenges.*

Index